Teen Doc Tells All

Your Most Personal Health Questions Answered by an Adolescent Medicine Specialist

Ilana Newman, MD

Newman Medical Enterprises, Inc.
NewmanMedicalEnterprises.com
Pembroke Pines, FL

i

Paperback ISBN: 978-0-9967508-06

Library of Congress Control Number 2015914794

First Edition
September 2015

Disclaimer Statement

Teen Doc Tells All covers a wide variety of teen health topics and is for educational and informational purposes only. The content is not intended to be a substitute for professional medical advice, diagnosis, or treatment. Always seek the advice of your physician or other qualified health provider with any questions you may have regarding your medical care or condition. No claims, promises, or guarantees about the completeness, accuracy, currency, content or quality of information contained in Teen Doc Tells All are made. You must not rely on this information as an alternative to medical advice from your doctor or other professional healthcare provider. If you think you may have a medical emergency, call your doctor or 9-1-1 immediately. Reliance on any information provided by Teen Doc Tells All is solely at your own risk. All advice given is intended to be discussed with your local doctor of choice.

Table of Contents

Sex Stuff

Preface

From 1999 to 2004, I wrote a sex and body column in Twist magazine each month. These were the same questions I answered from my patients each day – the kind of things teen girls don't feel comfortable asking their friends, parents, or pediatrician.

Over the years, I have met several regular readers of the column who told me how helpful and reassuring it was to read the questions and answers of other girls with similar concerns. Some even told me that if it wasn't for my advice, they might have done things that would have put their health and safety at risk.

Recently, a former reader of my column (who is now the mother of a young teen girl herself) expressed disappointment that there is no longer a similar source of this information for her daughter and her daughter's friends. This motivated me to dust off my old issues of Twist magazine and make this important advice widely available once again. Luckily, my contract stated that I retained the rights to what I wrote and could republish it.

Before you post a nasty review or fill my email box with complaints, I want you to know that I am fully aware these questions are repetitive. I noticed the same thing 15 years ago when receiving the reader questions from the magazine each month. But it was often the same way in my office, where I sometimes had to answer the same question half a dozen times in one day. Organizing the questions by topic makes the repetition much more obvious, but I felt that making the information easier to find was better than leaving you digging around for a particular answer. Also, some of the answers are more detailed or provide slightly different information, so I felt it was important to leave them all in. If you aren't looking for specific information, feel free to skip around when going through the book.

Other than some minor revisions (mostly removal of cheesy wording added by editors and updated medical information), the advice in this book is pretty close to my published answers from many years ago and is the same advice I would give to teen girls today. Other volumes in this series address questions about period problems and sex stuff.

While going through the process of reviewing and organizing the content for this book, I realized how much I enjoyed providing accurate and non-judgmental teen health advice. I know that these books will answer many of your questions, but I am sure you will have others or want more detailed information. To find out how you can submit your anonymous questions to me, Like the Teen Doc Tells All Facebook Page or go to TeenDocTellsAll.com . Check back regularly to see if your questions are answered like the ones in this book. I won't be able to get to them all, but I will make every effort to keep up as best I can.

This book was originally published as three separate ebooks – Teen Doc Tells All: Body Changes, Teen Doc Tells All: Period Problems, and Teen Doc Tells All: Sex Stuff.

Breast Distress

My left boob is bigger than my right one! I'm afraid people will think I'm a freak. Is there any way to fix this?

Body parts that come in pairs develop independently of the other side, which is why they aren't always the same size and shape. Most women have one breast that is larger than the other but usually there is less than a cup size difference. Large differences may be due to a development problem that happened before you were born or an injury to the chest area. Early in puberty, the difference may be more noticeable than when you're done developing, but size differences that are noticeable in older teens are unlikely to even out as you get older.

The easiest way to deal with an uneven bust is to add a little padding. Try borrowing some of the padding from another bra or use a removable bra pad. If the difference is a cup size or more, using a silicone bra insert may give you a less bumpy look. Silicone inserts can also be used in swimsuits because they don't soak up water. Some women decide to have plastic surgery to even things when they are adults, but most insurance companies consider this a cosmetic problem and won't cover the cost.

I always sleep on my stomach, but my friend says that will stop my boobs from growing! I know it sounds weird, but I'm pretty flat-chested, so I'm worried that she might be right. Is it true?

Sleeping on your stomach won't affect the size of your breasts or their shape. And wearing either regular bras or sports bras won't cause any damage. Your feet are in tight shoes all day and they keep growing, right?

Sleeping on your stomach can be a bit uncomfortable as sensitive breast tissue is developing, so you might find that you'll need to change your sleeping position in order to get a good night's sleep. Breasts continue to develop until your mid-twenties, so having a flat chest at your age doesn't forecast a flat chest in your future.

I'm 14 and my nipples are round and they stick out, so I can't go without a bra. But when I see older girls on TV, their nipples look normal. Will mine change as I get older?

Yes, your nipples, just like your breasts, will change over time. Most girls your age have nipples that are large and pointy – it kind of looks like they're just stuck onto your chest. But over the next few years, the breast tissue underneath will start to develop and the nipple will eventually become part of your overall breast shape. That's the stage that the older girls you see are at. Just like breasts, nipples come in all shapes and sizes. Right now, it's impossible for you to tell what your fully-developed breasts will look like or how your nipples will look in relation to them. Just give yourself some time to develop.

4

If you feel weird about how your breasts look, wear a padded bra so your nipples look more mature. The important thing is to be comfortable and not worry too much about your shape right now. In time, everything will fall into place.

The other day I felt a hard lump on the inside of my breast near the nipple. I've had my period for a year and I've never felt a lump before. Could I have cancer?

That is highly unlikely – breast cancer at your age is *extremely* rare. In fact, breast cancer is the least likely cause of your lump. So what *is* causing it? Breasts are made up of fat tissue, glands that produce milk, and fibrous tissue. Glands feel like pieces of rice under the skin and are easiest to detect under the areola (the dark skin around the nipple). But there are other kinds of larger lumps, called cysts and fibroadenomas, should be checked out by a doctor. Cysts are full of fluid, they can feel sore, and can get bigger or smaller during different times in your menstrual cycle. Fibroadenomas are solid, painless, and they don't change with your periods.
It can be scary when you first notice any lump, but don't worry – they're common and not usually anything to freak out about.

It's a good idea to do a breast self-exam every month, about a week after your period. Ask your doctor to show you how. That way, if you notice a lump you can tell your doctor how long it's been there and if it has become larger over time, which will help determine if you need any further tests.

I'm small chested, so I usually just wear a cotton tank top instead of a bra. But my friends say it's bad for me to take gym class without a bra on. Are they right?

No one *has* to wear a bra – from a medical standpoint. Of course, if you're wearing an outfit that's too revealing, going bra-free might earn you a few stares but it won't do any physical damage. A bra gives you support and keeps your breast from bouncing around when you move, but it's work for comfort and appearance, rather than medical reasons. Despite what you might have heard, bras don't stop breasts from sagging as you get older, especially if you are small-chested. It might make a slight difference in how *much* you sag, but unfortunately, gravity is going to win out no matter what.

Many women just feel more comfortable wearing a bra – especially while they're exercising. But if a tank top gives you enough support, tell your friends to mind their own business.

Is there anything I can do to make my boobs bigger?

Breasts may continue to grow until your mid-twenties, so there is no way to tell what size or shape they'll be when you're done developing. The size and shape of your breasts depend mostly on the genes you inherited from your parents, but being underweight can also make breasts smaller – after all, they're mostly fat.

If you are concerned with how your bust looks, try push-up or padded bras to help make your curves look smoother. Believe it or not, actresses and models sometimes use duct tape to create cleavage with low cut tops!

There are lots of ads promising lots of things when it comes to increasing breast size, but none of them have been proven to be safe and work. Breast enhancement pills or creams may contain hormones or herbs that can cause changes in your breasts and it's not known what effect they might have on breasts that are still developing. And there are no special exercises or devices that will make your breasts bigger.

My boobs are so big they bounce during gym and give me backaches 24/7. They're even starting to get saggy. How can I find relief?

Don't worry, there's plenty you can do. First, inspect your bra. Having the right one can make all the difference in terms of comfort. Weigh gain or loss, birth control pills and plain old puberty can all affect breast size, so the bra that fit you well last year may not be the right size for you now.

When buying bras, look for wide shoulder and back straps, which support large breasts much better than skinny straps. The back strap should also be in the right spot – on your middle back. If the back of the bra is creeping up on your shoulder blades, you need a larger size. Also, try bras on before you buy – and ask a salesperson for help if you need it. It may also be worth it to go to a place that specializes in women's underwear where an expert can measure you, tell you what size bra you really need, and help you select one that gives you proper support.

Women who experience severe pain from large breasts sometimes opt for breast reduction surgery. But like any operation, this comes with several risks, including complications due to the anesthesia, poor healing, and scars that could cause additional pain. So if your chest distress isn't improved with a better bra, discuss the option of surgery with your parents and doctor.

My best friend has huge boobs, and when we go out she always gets more attention than me. Is there anything I can to make my boobs seem bigger?

Sorry – there's not much you can to change the size of your chest. Upper body exercises like push-ups can build muscles in your chest and may make it seem fuller, but they won't make your breasts any bigger. And pills and creams that claim they can enlarge breasts may be ineffective or even dangerous.

Having big boobs can be a bummer – not all guys are subtle when they stare at your chest. Oversized breasts can even cause medical problems, like back and shoulder pain.

The good news is many guys don't think that breast size is important. Rather than focusing on increasing the size of your breasts, just be proud of who you are – confidence is way more eye-catching than cup size.

I just got boobs and I'm 20 years old!!! No, seriously! After years of being flat chested, I all-of-a-sudden have

breasts...and they're big ones, too! It's so bizarre though - why did I get them so late in the game? And is that normal?

Breast development can continue into your mid twenties. During your peak growing years, your body is concentrating on building bone, muscle, and skin to make you taller. If you have a big growth spurt and are on the thin side, your body doesn't have many calories left over for making curves – it can do that later when growing stops. And, since breasts are primarily made of fat, they take longer to fill out. That's also why you see so many tall guys in their late teens with skinny arms and legs who become less gangly when they start adding some bulk to their frames as they get older.

I noticed that my friends have brown circles around their nipples, while the area around my nipples is much pinker. Should I be worried?

Not at all. Just like other parts of the human body, the color, size, and shape of the areola (the area of skin around the nipples) varies from one woman to the next. Usually, the darker your all-over skin tone, the darker your areolas will be. They also tend to be pinker before puberty, then darken after your body starts producing more female hormones. Pregnancy and birth control pill use can also make areolas temporarily darker.

I think my nipples are inside out! I thought they were supposed to stick out, but mine don't. Is there something wrong with me?

Inverted nipples aren't that unusual – ten to twenty percent of women have them. And they are just as you describe them – when the tips point in instead of out. It's like the difference between bellybuttons that are "innies" and "outies" – it's just that "innies" are the less common variety when it comes to nipples. Some women have only one inverted nipple and some have both. You may notice that there is also a wide variety of sizes and colors of areolas – the rings of darker skin around nipples. That's just one more difference in breasts among women…

Other than how they look, inverted nipples are no different the non-inverted ones – they are just as sensitive, can be used for breastfeeding, and have nothing to do with the size or shape of your breasts. Young women with inverted nipples are usually born that way.

My friend says the Pill made her boobs grow. Is that true?

The truth is birth control pills *can* make your breasts a bit fuller. But they won't get so huge that you'll have to run out and buy bigger bras. In most cases, the change is pretty minimal. They get larger because the estrogen and progesterone in the Pill affect the breast tissue and cause your body to retain water.

Another side effect of the Pill can be weight gain. The hormones in the Pill can make you hungrier, so you'll gain weight – usually in the places that make women curvy: the chest, hips, and butt. But these changes aren't permanent and if you stop taking the Pill, your breasts will probably go back to their regular size. Getting larger breasts is not a good reason to go on the Pill, but for some it can be a nice bonus side effect.

My chest is pretty small, so I don't usually wear a bra. My friends do and they say that I'll get really saggy if I keep going braless. Is this true?

Here's the deal: There's absolutely no concrete evidence that wearing a bra will keep gravity from taking its toll on your chest as you get older and your skin becomes less elastic. And if you're smaller up top than your friends, you don't the same support they do.

For girls with larger chests, wearing a bra alleviates back and shoulder pain. Even if you're flat-chested, it's a good idea to wear a sports bra when you're working out or moving around a lot (whether or not you usually go braless) to keep your breasts from bouncing around too much. That will make your workout much more comfortable. Of course, years from now, if you do start to get a little saggy, a good bra will help give your breasts a lift. But aside from the support factor, there's nothing like a bra to give you great coverage underneath your favorite semi-sheer T-shirt - especially in a chilly environment if you want to avoid showing off your nipples.

Does wearing a tight bra or sports bra prevent your breasts from growing? I wear my sports bra all the time and I'm worried it's making me flat!

Relax! Sports bras might fit snuggly, but they can't affect how your breasts grow. So they're not keeping your from getting bigger. Your breasts will continue to grow whether you wear a tight bra, a loose bra, or no bra at all! Breast size is affected by a number of things, including the breast size of the women in your family and the amount of calories in your diet.

Sports bras are supposed to reduce the jiggle factor while working out, but they shouldn't be uncomfortable. Bras that are too tight can irritate the skin, causing red marks, indentations or skin infections. You might want to try to find a bra that you're totally comfortable in that still gives you the support you need.

I've noticed that my nipples cave in like my belly button and white stuff comes out of them. I'm really scared! Is something wrong?

What you are describing sounds like inverted nipples and galactorrhea (milk leaking from the breasts). Ten to twenty percent of women have inverted nipples and they are almost like the variation between belly buttons – some are "innies" and some are "outties." They are nothing to worry about unless an "outtie" nipple suddenly becomes inverted, which may be a sign of breast cancer in older women.

Birth control pills or pregnancy can stimulate milk production. But so can frequent stimulation of the nipples, so if you are trying to squeeze your inverted nipples out, this may be the cause. You should see a doctor for an examination and to have your level of prolactin (a hormone that stimulates milk production) checked. This type of hormone problem also may cause irregular periods and needs to be treated.

I have *no* boobs. The thing is I've already gotten my period and all of that, so does that mean they're not going to get any bigger?

Most women's breasts continue to develop into their early twenties, but there are some women who finish development earlier or later. The most drastic changes in breasts – going from a flat chest to needing a bra, happen before menstruation starts. But in the following years, the breasts slowing enlarge during the same time that other parts of your body get curvier. The final size of your breasts will mostly depend on what genes you inherited. Your weight is another factor because breasts are made mostly of fat, so being underweight can make your bust smaller than it should be based on your genes.

I've heard that sleep helps your body develop normally. But, uh, does it make *everything* develop? If I sleep ten hours a night, will it help my boobs grow faster?

I have never seen a study done to find out if sleep deprived teens are shorter or developing slower than they would be if they slept more. We may never find out the answer, because most teens – like most adults – don't get enough sleep. Some studies have shown that teens your age should get 12 hours of sleep each night – which is nearly impossible with all the homework and after school activities you're probably dealing with.

For the most part, rates of growth and development depend a lot on genes (if your mom was an early bloomer, you may be too) and good nutrition (starving bodies care more about staying alive than building bigger bones and muscles). Luckily, growth and development also happen together, otherwise teens could get pretty scary looking – imagine a short little boy with a full beard and mustache. This is why you've probably noticed that your girlfriends with larger chests are probably taller too. So, while getting enough sleep won't necessarily make your breasts larger, it may increase the chance that you'll be developing on schedule.

I have stretch marks around my nipple and they're really gross. Why do I have 'em? Will the marks every go away?

Don't worry. What's probably happened is that your breasts have grown a lot recently. And when rapid growth or weight gain occurs, the skin can't keep up so it stretches. These areas of thinned out skin, know as stretch marks, can appear anywhere on your body. Sometimes they're dark red or purple from the little blood vessels underneath the skin. After the skin stretches, it will slowly get thicker but the red marks can stay there. Over time, the marks will fade to a pink or shiny white color, kind of like a scar, but they'll never go away completely.
To make stretch marks less visible, use lots of moisturizer because dry skin makes them more obvious. Cocoa butter, shea butter or other greasy creams do the best job. Laser treatments are an option for really bad marks, but they're expensive and the results usually aren't great. For now, take comfort in the fact that lots of people have them – and they probably aren't as noticeable as you think.

I think I found a lump in my breast, and I'm so scared! Does that mean I have breast cancer? How can I tell for sure?

Breast cancer happens very rarely in someone your age, but that doesn't mean it never happens so you should get your lump checked out by a doctor. In general, the best time to examine your breast for lumps is a week after your period ends – at other times you might have some fluid retention that will make it harder to feel for lumps.

During your teens, it is very common for breasts to feel lumpy in general because the breast tissue is developing. This can feel like the breast tissue is all stuck together (like thick oatmeal) or you may be able to feel lots of little bumps (like cooked rice under the skin). Your breasts may also feel painful during your period because of the change in hormone levels and extra fluid.

If you find a lump in the same spot each time you examine your breasts, you should have a doctor examine you and possibly have an ultrasound test done to see if the lump is fluid-filled or solid. Mammograms aren't helpful in young women – the breast tissue is too thick and you can't see through them. In young women, these lumps are usually fluid filled cysts (which can often be drained with a needle) or a fibroadenoma (a non-cancerous lump that may continue to grow).

Ever since fourth grade, I've had to wear a bra. But I think they're uncomfortable, so I always wear a sports bra. Will this screw up my boobs?

There's no proof that wearing a certain type of bra – or not wearing one at all – can affect the size and shape of your breasts. You can wear sports bras anytime, but they can make your chest look flat, so most girls opt for traditional bras to make their chests appear fuller. If comfort is your main concern, sports bras are a great way to keep things snug and supported. Just steer clear of bras that are too tight, which can be uncomfortable and leave marks on your skin.

Can sleeping in your bra cause breast cancer? My friend says it's dangerous.

The rumor that bras actually cause breast cancer is silly. Several years ago, a study showed that there are more breast cancer cases in the United States, where most women wear bras, than in other countries where women go braless. But that doesn't mean that bras cause breast cancer because there are other big differences between women in different countries - like pollution, cigarette smoking, hormones and chemicals in foods, and stress levels. And don't worry about getting breast cancer from a too-tight bra either. If that were true, most women would have foot cancer from squeezing into tight shoes!

If you're worried that something you're doing might be dangerous, ask your doctor for her opinion. Of course, some habits - like smoking and excessive tanning - have been directly linked to cancer. But if you like a little support while you're sleeping, throw on a comfy bra and snooze away. You're not putting yourself at any risk.

My breasts aren't very big and neither are my mother's, but both my grandmothers are pretty well-endowed. Can I tell how big mine will get by looking at my relatives?

Unfortunately, there's no way to predict what your breast will look like until you're done developing. To some degree, breast size *is* inherited. But those genes can come from any one of your female relatives, so you have no way of knowing whose breasts yours will look like. Nutrition and exercise can also affect breast size. Because breasts are largely made up of fat, many female athletes and underweight models may have small busts even if their relatives have large ones. Being on the Pill can also temporarily enlarge breasts because of fluid retention and the effects of hormones.

Since your breasts may continue to grow until you're in your twenties, you'll have to wait and see if you turn out like your mom, grandmothers or somewhere in between. In the meantime, don't stress: Some girls develop much later than others, and breasts come in all shapes and sizes.

I've heard that you're supposed to check your breasts for lumps, but my boobs are lumpy all over! What's the deal? Am I deformed?

A self-breast exam isn't supposed to be a hunting expedition for any and all sorts of bumps – just the ones that need to be checked out further by a doctor. Breast tissue is lumpy, especially in young women – it can feel like a bowl of oatmeal that has been left sitting too long. While doing a self-breast exam, you may be able to feel the ducts that produce milk – they may feel like pieces of rice in all that other lumpiness. This may be more obvious during the two weeks before your period, when hormone levels affect the ducts.

Breast lumps that you need to tell your doctor about are those that are larger and don't feel like they're part of the surrounding breast tissue. They can have bumpy or smooth surfaces and can often be wiggled around a bit from side to side. In young women, most breast lumps aren't dangerous – they're usually fluid-filled cysts or solid fibroadenomas (a bit of breast tissue that decided to do its own thing). Cysts can be drained and fibroadenomas are either watched to see if they get bigger or they are removed with surgery. The risk of breast cancer goes up as a woman gets older, but there are some rare cases in women in their late teens and twenties, so make sure you tell your doctor about any lumps you're unsure about. Many women don't do self-exams the right way - ask your doctor to show you how.

I have these veins in my breasts that are really noticeable. Is this normal? How can I get them to go away?

It's totally normal to have visible veins on your breasts and upper chest area. A lot of light or fair-skinned people have veins you can see somewhere on their bodies. The veins on your breast are more noticeable because that skin is thinner since it had to stretch as your breasts developed.

Unfortunately, there's really no way to make the veins disappear. If they're really upsetting you or you're wearing something where they can be seen, you can cover them with waterproof makeup. Some makeup products are specifically designed for covering up birthmarks and spider veins on legs. These may work well, but you'll need a little practice to figure out how to apply it so it looks natural. Just remember that everyone has something that bugs them about their body, so try not to obsess about these veins. I'm sure you notice them more than anyone else who might see them.

I know it's normal to have different sized boobs, but what about nipples? Mine are different colors and different shapes! What's the deal?

Many people think we should have perfectly symmetrical bodies, but we aren't built that way. Just like eyes, hands, and feet, breasts don't match up one hundred percent. One nipple may be a different size, shape or color from the other. One or both nipples can also be inverted, pointing in like a belly button. Birth control pills, pregnancy and puberty can all affect how your nipples look due to the effects of hormones. So don't fret about your breasts. Unless you've noticed a recent change, everything is probably fine. But if you're really worried, have your doctor take a look.

I have little white dots on my nipples that look like white heads. What are they? Should I be concerned?

Don't worry. Those little white bumps are called sebaceous glands and you have them for a good reason. They produce a natural moisturizer to keep the circle of thin, dark skin surrounding the nipple (the areola) from drying out. Don't squeeze the glands to remove the white stuff - they're just going to fill up again and squeezing can lead to an infection. Sometimes these glands can get red or infected from being irritated by rough material rubbing against your skin. If you notice this kind of change, you should see a doctor to get checked out.

Don't freak out if your breasts don't look exactly like your friends' breasts. Some people have glands that are flat and others have glands that are raised, and the size, shape and color of the areola can vary greatly. Just try to remember that all breasts look different.

I noticed that my breasts get tender and lumpy right before I get my period, but the lumps go away once my period ends. Should I be worried?

Not at all. It's common for breasts to get a little lumpy, bumpy and sore around that time of the month. Some girls have fibrocystic breasts – the breast tissue contains tiny fluid filled cysts and firm connective tissue around them. Fibrocystic breasts are more sensitive to the hormone changes that happen each month, making them sore for several days before your period starts. The large bumps usually disappear between periods, but you may still be able to feel little gravel-like bumps under the skin in some places.

There are several things you can try to make coping with tender breasts during periods easier. Avoid super salty foods in the week before your period because they can cause increased water retention. Try cutting back on caffeine, from soda, coffee, or chocolate, to see if you notice an improvement. Exercising regularly during the week before your period may also help.

I always see those breast-enhancement pills advertised in magazines. Do they really work? I could definitely use some, uh, enhancement!

As a general rule, any pills or creams that only advertise in magazines or that you can only order online or by mail are suspicious. Any product that says it's natural but will cause a major change in your body is also questionable. These products often haven't been proven to work or safe and they aren't required to list all their ingredients or prove that each batch is the same, so you can't be sure about what you're taking.

Breast enhancement pills may contain hormones or herbs that can cause changes in your breasts and different brands have different ingredients. They probably can't make a big difference in breast size and any changes will go away if you stop taking them. Use of these products hasn't been proven to be safe and not lead to breast problems in the future. And it's not known what effect they might have on breasts that are still developing.

At your age, your breasts are far from being fully developed and it's no surprise that your chest doesn't seem adequate when you're still in the middle of puberty. Breasts may continue to grow until your mid-twenties, so there is no way to tell what size or shape they'll be when you're done. If you are concerned with how your bust looks, try a lightly padded bra that can help make your curves look smoother.

Sometimes I feel little lumps in my breast. I've never heard of a girl my getting breast cancer, but now I'm worried. Should I get them checked out?

First of all, breast cancer is extremely rare in teens and young adults. So why do you have lumps? As your breasts develop, they grow lots of new fat tissue and milk glands. Though some girls don't notice any change at all, others find that one or both of their breasts feel a little lumpy – almost like a beanbag – especially around the dark circle of skin near the nipple called the areola.

Most doctors recommend that you start having annual breast exams beginning at around age 18. This is also a good time to start doing monthly self-checks – you doctor will show you how. Though you're very unlikely to find anything serious, you'll get to know your breasts so you can spot changes later on. Of course, if you're worried about lumps and you're under 18, it's probably a good idea to see your doctor just to put your mind at ease.

Hair, Hair, Everywhere

I shaved my bikini area. Now that it's growing back it's really itchy. Anything I can do to help?

Sounds like you might have ingrown hairs. Shaving can irritate your skin, which may make it tough for hair (especially curly hair) to break back through the surface. Hairs that grow sideways through the skin become trapped, causing redness, itching and sometimes a small pimple-like infection.

Some safe shaving tips: When you use a new razor, dull the blade a bit by shaving your legs or underarms with it before heading to the bikini zone. Reduce irritation by lathering up with shaving cream or lots of sudsy soap.

If you do get an ingrown hair, don't operate on yourself! Instead, use an antibacterial soap on the area to prevent infection until the bump goes away. But if you notice it getting larger, more painful, or turning into a boil-like pimple, a doctor may need to help you out.

In the future, you might want to try waxing or using a chemical depilatory, but these non-razor methods also can cause irritation. Laser treatments can remove the hair, but they are kind of painful, require several treatments, are expensive and the results are often not permanent.

I've been losing a lot of hair lately. Is this normal? I'm afraid I'm going bald! What could be causing this?

Hair grows in cycles and everybody's hair has a pre-set maximum length before it falls out and a new hair grows. This is why people with long hair are more likely to complain that their hair is falling out – not to mention that long hairs make it look like more hair is lost when you see them in your brush or on the floor. Losing up to 100 hairs a day is normal, which is okay because the average person has several thousand hairs on their head.

Several things can make hair fall out abnormally fast. Chemotherapy treatments can make all hairs skip to the end of a growth cycle at once, so all hairs fall out at the same time. Some medical conditions may also cause hair loss, including problems with the thyroid gland and scalp infections. Estrogen makes hair grow extra fast and many women notice a significant amount of hair loss after having a baby or stopping birth control pills – this can be rather scary but it is temporary and most women don't see a difference in the amount of hair on their heads. Stress may cause hair loss but the results aren't usually as dramatic as other causes. There are also inherited forms of "female pattern" hair loss, which results in obvious thinning of the hair on the top of the head.

If you count up the hairs you lose each day and it's more than 100, see your doctor and find out if there is something that can be done. Don't bother with over-the-counter hair loss products without seeing a doctor first – they don't have rapid results and won't help if there is a medical reason for your hair loss.

Is it ok to cut or shave your pubic hair?

It is not dangerous to cut or shave your pubic hair – just be careful when you do it. Like the hair anywhere else on your body, pubic hair grows back. Skin in the pubic area has more sweat glands than in other places and this can make you feel pretty itchy as hair grows back.

There are different ways to get rid of unwanted hair down there and every woman figures out what works best for her. The most common method is shaving with water and lots of soap or shaving cream. This will soften the hair and keep the skin moisturized to help prevent razor burn. Don't use a brand new razor or apply too much pressure on the razor handle. Irritated skin after shaving can lead to ingrown hairs because curly pubic hairs don't always grow straight up through the skin. Ingrown hairs can become infected but most of the time they just cause ugly red bumps. If the red bumps get large, painful or look like pimples, have a doctor check them out.

Trimming the hair with scissors doesn't cause ingrown hairs because the hairs still stick out of the skin. Hair doesn't grow back as fast when removed with depilatory creams, but a lot of people find the chemicals irritating or the smell unbearable. Waxing also lasts longer than shaving, but it can be painful and expensive if done at a salon.

I have dark hairs on my face, my chest, and even my stomach. What's wrong with me? How can I get rid of it?

First of all, there's nothing wrong with being hairy. Most people have hair in places they wish they didn't, guys and girls alike! Some people have thin, light hair and others have thick, dark hair –it depends mostly on your ethnic background. If you also have bad acne or periods which come every few months you could have a hormonal imbalance which should be checked out by a doctor. Otherwise, I wouldn't freak – there are lots of fixes for hairy situations. Bleaching creams can lighten hair so it's less noticeable, but you need to do it every few weeks. Shaving, depilatory creams and waxing remove hair temporarily, but you have to deal with itchy stubble as it grows back. Electrolysis and laser hair removal are more permanent solutions, but they can be expensive and require multiple treatments. You may want to experiment and see what works for you.

Help! I've got hair on my nipples! Does that mean I'm a freak?

No, it doesn't. Body hair can develop almost anywhere during puberty! Your body's just creating hormone, which stimulate hair growth in places other than your private parts – armpits, arms, legs, face, stomach, and yes, your nipples.
Of course, realizing that hairy nipples are normal probably doesn't make you any happier about them. But because the skin around your nipples is sensitive, you have to be careful about getting rid of nipple hairs. Shaving or trimming the hairs is less likely to cause irritation or skin infections than plucking or

waxing. Depilatory creams are usually too strong for thin nipple skin and can leave you with a big rash. Just don't stress too much about it – chances are your friends are freaking out about the same thing!

I shaved my bikini line to get ready for swimsuit season. But now I have these horrible red bumps down there, and it itches like crazy. Did I give myself some kind of weird rash?

Yikes – razor burn! Those little red bumps that appear after shaving may be annoying, but they're rarely anything to worry about. The skin around each hair follicle can get irritated and, as the hairs grow back, they can't get through the swollen skin. So they grow under the skin, making little itchy bumps.

There are a few tricks to make razor burn less likely. Make sure to use lots of shaving cream or soapy water and never shave dry skin. When you buy a new razor, chose one with a lubricating strip so it will irritate your skin less and shave your legs with it first, so that the sharp blades won't scrape the sensitive skin around your bikini line. And because a tight bikini or salt water can irritate freshly shaved skin, try shaving the night before you plan a day at the pool or beach. You skin will feel smooth and stay itch-free in no time!

My friend told me that dyeing my hair can cause cancer. Is that true?

The connection between hair dye and cancer was first reported many years ago but it hasn't been proven. Some studies have shown that women who dye their hair are more likely to get certain kinds of cancer but other studies didn't find the same results. This is why hair dye is still sold and there is no warning label on packages.

Unfortunately, that's how it goes with scientific research – each study only gives us a piece of the puzzle and it may take long time before we know for sure if something causes a disease or cancer. If you are still concerned that coloring your locks today may cause problems tomorrow, there are some things you can do to try to be safer. Permanent dyes are the biggest cancer-causing suspects, so you might want to try semi-permanent products that fade out in a month or two. Darker colors may also be riskier than lighter shades. And the studies that linked hair dyes and cancer found that the risk goes up the more you use them, so you might want to wait until some gray hairs pop up before you start using hair dye on a regular basis.

Help! My hormones are out of control. Lately, I've noticed hair in really strange places, like on my arm, my upper lip, and even my stomach. Why is this happening and what can I do to get rid of it?

Body hair starts developing ALL over during puberty. This is due to hormone stimulation of hairs in places in addition to your private parts – armpits, arms, legs, face, nipples, and stomach. Hair is very sensitive to your level of testosterone (which all women have, but less of it than men do). In women, these hairs are usually thinner and less dark than the hairs in on your head. When this hair starts growing during puberty, most women start experimenting with ways to remove it.

The amount of body hair you'll have depends on two things – genes and hormones. If the women in your family tend to be on the hairy side, you're likely to wind up the same way. If you notice a sudden increase in the amount of body hair after puberty or think you are more hairy than other people in your family, see a doctor because it could be due to a hormone imbalance. The doctor should check your hormone levels and examine the amount and locations of the hairs.

Electrolysis is a permanent method of hair removal, but it's expensive, slow, and painful. Laser treatments can remove hair but the effects may not be permanent, it's expensive, and it works best in people with light hair and dark skin. More traditional forms of hair removal, like shaving, waxing, and depilatory creams, are cheaper but the effects don't last as long.

"Down There" Despair

I have this stuff in my underwear that looks like mucus. My periods started 7 months ago and I've only had them three times. What is this stuff? Is this normal?

No one tells young women that it's normal to have a discharge from the vagina every day after puberty starts kicking in. The color (when wet) can be white, gray, clear, or light yellow and it may have a faint odor. Based on changes in hormone levels during a monthly cycle, it can be watery or very stretchy.

Vaginal discharge can be annoying, so here are some tips on coping with it. Wear all cotton panties (not just ones with cotton in the crotch) and don't wear underwear while you sleep. The more air that circulates down there, the less discharge you'll notice. Wear panty liners only when you have your period for the same reason – the plastic backing doesn't let air in. Wash your private parts just once a day with mild soap, using only your hands (no washcloth, sponge or net). Don't scrub or wash inside the vagina – this can cause irritation and make you have even more discharge. And don't douche – it only upsets the normal balance inside the vagina (which is "self-cleaning") and can lead to funky discharges.

What exactly *is* a yeast infection?

Yeast is a type of fungus that is normally found in low levels on your skin, in your intestines, and in your vagina, just like many kind of bacteria. Usually it's not a problem and you'd never know it's there until something changes its normal environment, giving it a chance to multiply and cause problems.

A yeast infection is pretty much the same thing as a baby's diaper rash – an overgrowth of yeast causing a red irritation down below. The yeast causes a lot of thick, white vaginal discharge – it doesn't smell bad but the itching can be unbearable. Most yeast infections are cured quickly with creams you can buy at any drugstore. But if you've never had one before, it's important that you see a doctor first to make it is only a yeast infection. Once you've had one, you'll be able to recognize it if happens again and you can try treating it yourself. There are also prescription medications that will clear up a yeast infection if it doesn't respond to over-the-counter medications.

The most common cause of yeast infections in women is antibiotic medication, which kill off bacteria everywhere in your body, giving the yeast a chance to multiply and cause problems. If this happens to you all the time, you may want to buy a tube of yeast infection cream when you pick up your antibiotic prescription. Similar to the type of yeast used to bake bread, the yeast on and inside your body loves to grow in warm and wet areas. Changing out of wet swim suits, wearing cotton panties, not wearing underwear at night can also help keep the area down there drier and may help prevent yeast infections.

I have to go to the gyno, and I'm freaking out about getting a Pap smear! I'm totally embarrassed. Why do I need one?

Once you've started having sex, it's important to have Pap smears done so you *know* you're healthy But don't worry, they aren't scary. It may seem weird having your doctor getting so up close and personal with your private parts, but no need to be embarrassed – she does this for a living! Your doctor will collect cells from your cervix to test them for cancerous or abnormal cells. Some girls feel minor cramping, but it's pretty painless. You'll also get tested for gonorrhea and chlamydia, which are sexually transmitted infections. Your doctor will also do an internal exam to make sure the size and shape of your ovaries and uterus are normal. The whole visit is over in about 15 minutes, so don't sweat it!

I think I have a vaginal odor problem. I tried douching, but it didn't help. Is something wrong with me? What can I do?

Funky odors down below can happen for several reasons. Most people don't realize that everyone's genital area has more sweat glands and bacteria than other skin and gets pretty stinky. You should wash "down there" once a day with a mild soap. Washing too often can cause irritations or rashes. And no scrubbing - use just your hands gently because a washcloth or sponge can be too rough on the delicate skin. Women shouldn't try to wash inside the vagina or douche. The high level of acid in a vagina keeps things normal, but douche or soap inside the vagina makes things less acid, leading to funky discharges and itching from overgrowth of bacteria and yeast. Sleeping without underwear, wearing all cotton panties, and changing out of wet bathing suits and sweaty clothes after workouts can help keep the balance by improving air circulation below the waist.

Some STDs can cause bad odors, along with itching, painful urination, or an abnormal discharge. If you've had sex, have a doctor check you out.

Help - I think something's wrong! One of the lips of my vagina is way longer than the other. Does that mean there's a problem down there?

Eyes, breasts, hands, feet – if a body part comes in pairs, there's a good chance you'll get two different sizes. This is because each half of the pair develops on its own. Most of the time, the difference isn't even noticeable. But just like your breasts can vary by a cup size or more, your labia (the lips of your vagina) can be visibly uneven. (There are actually two sets of labia – the outer labia majora and inner labia minora.)

Here's the good news: There is nothing wrong with you! There are plastic surgeons who will operate to correct the appearance of labia, but this is expensive, painful, and really not necessary because no one sees this part of your body in public.
The only time you need to worry is if one of your labia suddenly increases in size - this could be a sign of an infection and should be checked out by a doctor.

I have really bad vaginal discharge - so bad that I have to wear a pad every day to school. Is there anything I can do to stop it? I am only 13 and never had sex. Please help me!

Believe it or not, your best bet is to ditch the pads – the plastic backing doesn't let air circulate and can actually make discharge worse. High temperatures, perfumes, douches, and bubble baths also change the acid levels in your vagina, which can cause abnormal discharges.

It's normal to have discharge every day, and the amount and thickness changes with different hormone levels throughout the month. Unless it itches, smells bad, or looks dark yellow or green, it's totally normal. Wear cotton underwear during the day and sleep without underwear at night - it allows air to circulate and may reduce the amount of discharge.

My friend told me that I should squat instead of sitting down when I use a public bathroom because I can catch a yeast infection from a dirty toilet seat. Is she right?

Despite what you might have heard, it's hard to catch *anything* from a toilet seat. When you sit down properly on a toilet, it's just your thighs that touch the seat, so to catch something you'd really have to wiggle all over it. Plus, most of the things people worry about catching – yeast infections, HIV and sexually transmitted infections – don't live very long on cold, non-living surfaces. Yeast infections aren't usually spread from one person to another like that. They develop internally when your body's balance of yeast and bacteria gets out of whack.

Yeast is a type of fungus that is always present in the vagina in small amounts. When women douche, take antibiotics, use scented tampons, hang out in a wet bathing suit for hours or even get stressed out, the normal vaginal environment is disturbed and the good bacteria become fewer. This lets the yeast multiply, causing an itchy, thick, white discharge – a yeast infection. If you've had a yeast infection before and think you have one again, an over-the-counter remedy should do the trick. If it doesn't work or if you're not completely sure that you have yeast infection, have a doctor check you out.

I was really itching down there and having a lot of white discharge, so I tried an over-the-counter yeast infection cream. But it's still itching like crazy. I've never had sex so I know I don't have an STI. What should I do?

Sounds like you should talk to your doctor. If you have a yeast infection, a three- or seven-day vaginal yeast infection treatment that contains an applicator or suppository, usually does the trick. So, if you were careful about following the directions and the itching still hasn't stopped, you may need a stronger prescription medication.

It's also possible that you have a different kind of infection, like bacterial vaginosis, which develops when your vagina's delicate balance of bacteria gets messed up. Lots of people mistake this condition for a yeast infection because the symptoms can be similar, but bacterial vaginosis has a funky smelling discharge which is thinner and grayish (as opposed to the white, thick, no odor discharge with a yeast infection). Don't worry, though. While both problems are minorly unpleasant, they're common and totally treatable. Your best bet: Get yourself to the doctor. Once she figures out what's causing all that itching, she'll put you on the road to recovery.

I have all these little bumps near my vagina. I've never had sex or even fooled around with a guy, so it can't be an STI, right? So what is it?

There are several times of little bumps in the area around a vagina that can be normal. The most common type is ingrown hair, which can be skin colored, red, or even have a whitehead like a pimple. Sometime you can actually see the curled up hair under the skin. These kinds of bumps are found in the area where hair grows and can be caused by friction from underwear that is too tight or from shaving. You can even get little ingrown hairs on your butt where you sit!

Other kinds of bumps that can be found around the vagina are tiny glands in the skin that keep the sensitive area down there moisturized. These bumps look like the bumps on chicken skin and are also found on areolas (the dark skin around nipples). Friction from tight underwear can also cause these bumps to get bigger or red because the openings to the glands get blocked. But don't scratch or squeeze them – this will only make the irritation worse and can lead to infection. The best way to deal with them is to put a washcloth with warm water on that area. If these bumps are in the area where the skin touches the crotch of your underwear, stop wearing thongs, get underwear a size larger, and try sleeping without underwear at night to give your skin a break.

What exactly is a Pap smear? One of my friends just had one, and when she told me, I had no idea what she was talking about. Is it painful?

A Pap smear is a test for abnormal cells on the cervix. It's named after the guy who invented it, Dr. Papanicolaou, and now fewer women die of cervical cancer because of this little test. Women should have a pap smear at least once a year, beginning when they first have sex. The main causes of cancer of the cervix are smoking cigarettes and sex (mostly because of the human papillomavirus, also known as HPV). There is now a vaccine that reduces the chance of cervical cancer by protecting you from the most dangerous types of HPV.

Pap smears don't hurt. After the doctor uses a speculum to look at your cervix, and a brush (like a miniature broom) touches the cervix to get some cells for the test. You'll feel it touching you and you might also feel some mild cramps, but that's it. The cells are sent to a lab so a pathologist can check them under a microscope. The doctor will also test you for some STIs and your ovaries and uterus are also examined during the pelvic exam. Schedule your appointment for a time when you won't be on your period and don't have sex or put anything in your vagina for two days ahead of time. And don't stress about the exam – almost everyone has the same test done every year.

I have this whitish stuff that kinda smells on my underwear. It's there almost every day. Should I be worried?

You know how some ovens are "self-cleaning?" Well, the vagina is self-cleaning too. Believe it or not, it is normal to have a discharge from your vagina every day. Normal discharge can be white, gray, clear or light yellow and might have a faint odor.

Sometimes the discharge is annoying, so here are some ways to cope: Wear all-cotton panties (not just ones with cotton in the crotch) which let your skin breathe. Wear panty liners only when you have your period (not every day) and use ones that are unscented. Wash your private parts once a day with mild soap, but don't scrub or wash inside the vagina with soap – this can make discharges smell worse. The best advice – sleep without underwear for maximum air circulation at night!

What is a yeast infection? I have itching down there sometimes. Do I have one?

You might not know it, but yeast is a kind of fungus that is *always* present in the vagina. Under normal circumstances, it's kept in check by good bacteria so it doesn't irritate or itch. But sometimes the yeast can grow out of control and cause an infection. This can happen for lots of reasons – taking birth control pills or antibiotics, taking bubble baths, having an increased amount of stress, or sweating excessively. All of these things can change the environment in the vagina so that yeast multiply and take over. And you don't have to be sexually active to get a yeast infection – even babies get diaper rash versions.

So how can you tell if you have a yeast infection? You will notice an itchy, thick, white vaginal discharge. But unlike other vaginal infections, the discharge from a yeast infection doesn't smell bad. If it smells at all, it's usually a slightly sweet odor or a little like bread. It can be confusing since not all discharge or itching means you have a yeast infection. That's why you should get checked out by a doctor who can make a diagnosis and prescribe the right treatment. Yeast infections are common and, once you know how to identify them, you can treat them yourself with medications available at the pharmacy without a prescription.

I have a piece of flesh that hangs below the lips of my vagina – you can actually see it when I stand up. Is there something wrong with me?

Unless you've had a major trauma to your private parts, you're most likely completely normal. Here's a guide to what you might be seeing: Between the labia majora (the big, outer lips) are the labia minora (the thinner, inner lips), which can be longer, shorter, or the same length as the bigger ones. You may be seeing the inner lips peeking out – or your clitoris, which sits between the labia minora. You can get familiar with the area yourself by taking a look. Lie on your back under a good light and hold a small mirror down there. It might seem freaky, but it'll help you get to know your body better. Still have questions? Your doctor has heard them all before and she'll be more than happy to check you to and reassure you that you're normal.

I think I have zits down there! I get these little red bumps that look like pimples, and I don't know what's causing them. How can I get rid of them?

Tiny bumps that are only at hair follicles (where the hairs come through the skin) are probably a condition called folliculitis. It can happen anywhere there's hair on your body and it usually starts because something is irritating the skin. Clothes that are too tight, scratching your skin, or razor burn are common causes. Sometimes the little bumps get infected and get very red or turn into whiteheads and need to be treated with antibiotics.

If your bumps down below are where you're shaving, using plenty of soapy water, not pressing hard with your razor, and not using a brand new razor (it's too sharp) on your bikini line may help. Try not to scratch even though it gets itchy when the hairs grow back. Warm compresses may help clear up the bumps you have now but if you have whiteheads or the bumps turn into open sores, see a doctor.

I peeked at myself down there and I don't think I'm normal. It was all dark and there wasn't a lot of hair. How is it supposed to look down below when you're 14?

Believe it or not, there's no "normal" way to look down there. Female private parts are very different from woman to woman. The color, texture and amount of pubic hair varies with each person. How your lady parts look depends mostly on your ethnic background and they probably look like those of the other women in your family.

In general, the outer lips are usually covered with hair and may be darker than the surrounding skin. The inner lips aren't as thick as the outer ones and they're hairless and more pink and sensitive than skin in other areas. Just remember that every woman is different – and there's no such thing as normal or not. So unless you have pain or symptoms that make you think need medical attention, there's no reason for you to worry.

I'm confused about douching. Some of my friends do it but my mom says it's not good for you. Should I do it?

Many girls see ads for douche products on television and laugh – but then wonder if douching is something they're supposed to do. Absolutely not! Women don't need to douche because vaginas are self-cleaning. You know that vaginal discharge you see on your underwear? That's evidence of this natural cleansing process.

Not only is douching not necessary, it can actually cause problems. By rinsing out the good bacteria in your vagina and making the environment less acidic, you could cause an infection like bacterial vaginosis or a yeast infection. Some women start douching because they have one of these problems already, but douching can make matters worse. Plus, the perfumes in douches can be very irritating. And if you're sexually active, douching may make it easier for some sexually transmitted infections (STIs) to infect your cervix or cause them to speak into a serious case of pelvic inflammatory disease. The bottom line; steer clear of douches.

I'm not due for my period yet this month, but I have this thick, clear discharge. Is that normal?

Every girl has normal vaginal discharge that starts when she hits puberty. It's just one of the ways the vagina cleans itself. Depending on your hormone levels and where you are in your cycle, the discharge can be either gooey and clear (kind of like phlegm) or thin and clumpy. Either way, it's usually clear, white or light yellow. (Check the color when it's wet - it will appear darker and scarier when it dries and after your period when it could be brownish for a few days.) If your discharge is an unusual color, starts to itch, or smells bad, have your doctor check you out to make sure you don't have an infection that needs treatment.

I love wearing thong underwear, but I've heard that they can be bad for your health. Is that true?

Thongs aren't really a health hazard, but they are more likely to cause some problems than other types of underwear. Because a thong's crotch area is narrow, it's more likely to cause skin irritation from constantly rubbing against sensitive areas. Wearing thongs that are the right size and made of cotton may help, but the only way to avoid this problem is if the edges of the crotch area reach your inner thighs on both sides. Another problem sometimes associated with wearing thongs is bacterial vaginosis (BV), which is an overgrowth of stinky bacteria due to a decrease in the acid level in the vagina. Unprotected sex, douching, and tight-fitting underwear/pants that keep the area

42

down there hot and sweaty all can lead to BV. Alternating your thongs with regular underwear, wearing cotton thongs, and not wearing underwear at night may help reduce your chances of having to deal with BV.

I read somewhere that eating too much bread can cause yeast infections. Can food really affect that kind of stuff?

You might think eating something made with yeast (bread) makes you prone to yeast infections (those down-there problems that can cause from itching and thick, lumpy discharge). But they really happen when your vagina's normally low yeast level gets disrupted and starts to multiply out of control.

Before you think about banning bread from your diet, consider this: the yeast in bread gets killed during baking. There has never been any real proof that bread (or anything you eat for that matter) causes yeast infections. Similarly, eating yogurt (though really good for you and contains a bacteria similar to the one in vaginas) may not prevent yeast infections as well as some people think. The one food that might make yeast infections more likely is sugar. Yeast eats sugar and starts multiplying faster than usual.

The Skin You're In

I had a cold sore on my lip, and my friend said that means I have herpes. Is that true?!

It's true that cold sores are caused by the herpes virus but don't panic. Having oral herpes doesn't mean you have the genital kind. You may have caught it years ago when a relative with a cold sore gave you a big, wet kiss. Or you could have got it from smooching your boyfriend.

Once you're infected, the herpes virus stays in your body and can cause sores any time your immune system isn't working perfectly (like if you're sick or stressed). The sores usually heal after five to seven days with no scars left behind. But remember: While most people think herpes is only contagious when a sore is visible, you're actually just as likely to spread the virus to someone else *before* one appears. The area may be tingly for a day before an outbreak but often people have no idea when one is about to pop out.

When you see sores or think one is coming, wash your hands often, don't touch your cold sores, and avoid lip-to-skin contact with anyone until the outbreak is over. Oral sex is also a no-no, since you can transmit oral herpes to the genital area when cold sores come in contact with private parts. There are two types of the virus - herpes simplex virus I, which usually causes cold sores on the mouth, and herpes simplex virus II, which usually causes sores on the genitals, but both forms could be spread from either area.

There are topical creams you can buy without a prescription that may help outbreaks heal faster. If your cold sore outbreaks happen frequently, see your doctor who can test the sore to determine what virus is causing it and may prescribe a daily medication to prevent the outbreaks.

A couple years ago I started getting stretch marks on my hips and breasts. I'm not heavy but they're keeping me from wearing short skirts. Is there anything I can do to minimize them without surgery?

The bad news about stretch marks is that there isn't much you can do about them. The good news is that they tend to get much lighter with time. Stretch marks happen when growth or weight gain happens faster than skin can grow, so the skin has to stretch. These areas of thinned-out skin can appear anywhere on your body and also happen in guys. Stretch marks can be red or purple because the thinner skin shows the blood vessels underneath. Just like with a scar, the skin eventually returns to a normal thickness and the color lightens up, but the marks never go away completely.

Using lots of moisturizer on your skin helps reduce the dryness that makes stretch marks more noticeable. The greasier the lotion or cream, the better it will work. Laser treatments are available, but they are expensive and the results usually aren't great. Waterproof makeup that is made to cover up scars and burns can help disguise stretch marks until they fade.

I know this is totally gross, but I have acne on my butt! Can I just use the same stuff I put on my face back there?

Acne is not limited to your face - it can pop up on chests, necks, backs, and butts. Treating acne that's not on your face is kind of tricky because it's not easy to see where you're trying to put acne medication. Also, most acne products come in tiny containers that are too small for using on larger areas of skin.

Keeping your skin clean is the key, so use an antibacterial soap in the shower. Be careful not to rub hard with a towel when drying off – that will only irritate your skin more and make breakouts worse. Washes or soaps containing salicylic acid or benzoyl peroxide can be used if breakouts get out of control. You can treat specific spots with the same drying pimple creams that you use on your face if needed. And the rule about no touching/scratching/picking goes for your body as well as your face.

Acne on your butt or other areas that often get rubbed by clothing may not really be true acne. Folliculitis (inflammation of the hair follicles) is common in people who ride bikes, wear tight clothing, or who spend lots of time sitting – it happens because the skin is constantly irritated and bacteria on the skin cause little pimple-like infections. If you have bumps over a large part of your butt, you should see a doctor and find out if you have folliculitis and need antibiotics to get it under control.

My boyfriend gave me a hickey and I didn't even feel it. What are those things anyway? They look gross!

Hickeys are basically like bruises, but unlike bruises elsewhere on your body, everyone knows how you got that mark on your neck. They are caused by little tears in the blood vessels in the skin and blood starts to leak out under the skin. This is also why they can sometimes be painful.

Under normal circumstances, the biggest problem with a hickey is covering it up. The best thing is to put some ice on it and hide it with a turtleneck or makeup. Like other bruises, you won't be able to make it go away quickly - you'll have to wait for it to slowly change color and fade away. If you find yourself hiding your hickeys after every date with your guy, tell him to ease up on the suction power.

I have acne all over my chest. My mom says it's from playing basketball. Is she right? Or should I see a dermatologist?

Zits can pop up almost anywhere, and since your chest has a lot of oil-producing glands, it's definitely pimple prone. When you play sports, your clothes can rub against your skin and irritate it, so sweat and dirt can clog your pores. But that definitely doesn't mean you should stop playing basketball. Just remember to shower right after playing and change out of your sweaty clothes.

You may also want to try an acne-fighting body wash when you shower. Products with salicylic acid may help for mild cases, but benzoyl peroxide will work better although it can cause irritation and redness. If you're taking care of your skin but still battling breakouts, talk to your doctor the next time you go for a check up. She'll be able to give you a prescription acne medication or may refer you to a dermatologist.

I had a major growth spurt this year and gained about 15 pounds. I'm not worried about the weight – I'm just happy I finally have curves! - but I started noticing stretch marks on my hips and my butt. What causes them, and is there anything I can do to make them go away?

When your body grows faster than you can make enough skin, the skin thins out in some areas, leaving stretch marks. They can happen if you have a sudden weight gain or fast growth spurt. That's why many tall guys have horizontal stretch marks on their backs! The stretch marks start out a reddish or darker color because the thinner skin shows the blood vessels underneath, but they become lighter with time. They may never disappear completely but dry skin makes them easier to see, so use a moisturizer.

My boyfriend says that my lips are really scratchy when we kiss. No matter what I do, I just can't make them moist. Help!

Scratchy smackers, huh? It happens to all of us. The skin on the lips, unlike the skin on most other parts of your body, doesn't have glands that keep it naturally moisturized. That's why cold weather, licking your lips, and even kissing can really dry you out. But there are a few things you can do: For starters, wear lip balm year-round (the greasier, the better) and use one with SPF 15 or higher sunblock if you're out in the sun. Reapply it often, over and under lipstick, after a makeout session, and before you go to bed at night. And if you tend to lick or bite your lips, kick that habit right away! You'll be more kissable in no time.

Is tanning really all that bad for me?

All of your sun exposure over your lifetime adds up and will come back to haunt you later on. This may be hard to believe when the worst damage you usually see is some peeling with a burn. Tanning is the way your skin tries to protect itself from ultraviolet rays, but there is no level of sun exposure that is absolutely safe, including tanning beds. Sun damage increase your risk of getting skin cancer but it also makes skin look old while you're still young.

Blondes and redheads with light colored eyes have skin that's more likely to become sun damaged and having lots of moles increases the risk of melanoma (a type of skin cancer). In the past, skin cancers appeared later in life, but more cases are being diagnosed in late teens and young adults in the past few years, probably due to more sun exposure at an earlier age and use of tanning beds.

If applied correctly, self-tanning products can fool almost anyone. They don't provide any protection against burning, so you still need to use sunblock. Make sure your sunblock protects against both UVA and UVB rays and that you reapply it after swimming or sweating.

I always get cold sores on my lips, and my friend told me it's probably herpes. But I've never even kissed a guy! I couldn't possibly have herpes, right?

Herpes simplex viruses cause little fluid-filled blisters to appear in a cluster and burst, leaving a painful ulcer that slowly dries up. The virus hides out in nerves and creates new outbreaks in the same area when your immune system is weakened by stress, poor diet, or illness (which is where the name "cold sores" come from).

The location of the blisters or the particular strain of virus (HSV-1 or HSV-2) isn't as important as knowing that it's very contagious and spread by skin-to-skin contact. Your case is a good example – you've never had sex but someone, probably a relative, with herpes on his or her lips kissed you. This is why it's important that when you have a cold sore that you avoid kissing anyone and touching your eyes or other parts of your body after touching your lips. And it's possible for herpes to be spread from mouth to genitals (or vice versa) during oral sex. Herpes infections are most contagious before the blisters appear (many people report the area gets numb or tingly a few days before an outbreak) and until they completely heal. The virus is present in low levels at other times and could still be spread but the risk is much lower.

More Than Enough of the Other Stuff

I brush my teeth every morning before I leave for school, but as soon as I get to homeroom, I can tell that I have bad breath. I'm so self conscious! Please Help!

Funky breath leaving a bad taste in your mouth? It happens to all of us. The stink is from normal bacteria in our mouths that are breaking down leftover food particles. This is why everyone's breath is especially rank when we wake up - those hours of not much saliva and no swallowing lets the bacteria have parties in our mouths.

If you skip breakfast, the digestive juices and acid in your stomach build up and can cause burping, bad breath, or a stomach ache. Feeling nervous about a test or class presentation may make your breath even worse, so make sure to eat something before going to school. Starchy foods are the best things to soak up the acid in your stomach, like toast, cereal, or crackers. If you don't have time for breakfast before school, keep granola bars or a breakfast bar in your bag to snack on.

Brushing your teeth helps, but it's only the first step. Try brushing your tongue too and using dental floss to get rid of the food between teeth. You can also try antiseptic mouthwash to kill some of the stinky bacteria. If you haven't been to a dentist in a while, make an appointment for a cleaning and check up - you may have a cavity without knowing it. Your dentist may have other suggestions for dealing with your bad breath if nothing else seems to work.

I want to get in shape, and I read somewhere that you should lift weights. But my friend says it'll actually make me gain weight! Is she right?

It's true that muscle weighs more than an equal amount of fat. But the main goal of weight lifting isn't weight loss – it's to increase muscle tone and definition. That's why using a scale alone can't determine if someone is in shape or not. Using body mass index (BMI) calculations that use height and weight and calculating percent body fat is a much better way to determine if someone is fit or fat.

Exercising with light weights is good for almost everyone and can help increase the strength of bones in addition to toning muscles. There is some concern that lifting heavy weights before your body finishes growing may stunt your growth, but there is not science to support this risk. Heavy weight lifting does increase the risk of injuries like torn ligaments and tendons or damaged joints in growing bodies, so it would be wise to hold off on serious bodybuilding training until you're over age 18.

Whenever something goes slightly wrong, I feel miserable and dwell on it for days. I think it's just the blues but my mom's afraid I might suffer from depression. How can I tell the difference?

Mood swings may feel a lot like depression, but there are ways to tell if you're suffering from something more serious than a simple case of the blues. If you had a bad day and you're feeling bummed, that's normal. But if you're sad and irritable for more than two weeks or you lose interest in activities that you usually enjoy and withdraw from your friends, you may be suffering from depression. You should also be looking for big changes in sleeping habits or appetite, feeling like you're moving in slow motion, having no energy, feeling worthless or guilty for no reason, and having thoughts about death or hurting yourself. If any of these apply, *please* talk to your parents and doctor right away. Depression is a medical problem that may get worse without help and can be treated with counseling and medication.

I get tingly when my boyfriend kisses me in weird places like my earlobes. It there a medical reason for this? I told my friends about my secret turn-on spots and they started ragging on me.

Those tingles are your body's natural way of telling you that you're into your guy. Everyone has super-sensitive spots called erogenous zones. The most obvious one is your genital area, but those feel-good zones are all over – often in surprising places like the neck, ears, cheeks, and fingers. Your body is physiologically reacting to being touched and complicated chemical reactions involving nerves and hormones lead to those sensations. But your mood and the person doing the touching play a huge role in whether it makes you feel happy or annoyed. After all, you're more likely to shiver in delight when your boyfriend nibbles your ear than when your dog plants a wet kiss there!

I'm 16 years old, but I'm only 4'11" *so* much shorter than all of my friends! How do I know if I'm done growing? Is there any way for me to get taller?

A person's final height usually is somewhere between their mother's and father's heights and you can't do much about short parents. A shorter than expected height can be due to several things, such as poor nutrition, a genetic disorder, or a hormonal problem. In women, the biggest growth spurts happen before periods start, although some women continue to grow slowly until they are about twenty years old.

When your doctor checks your height at annual checkups, it's not just so you know how tall you are. Each of those measurements is put on a piece of graph paper, called a "growth curve" to see if you're growing at a normal rate. If someone's growth has suddenly stopped or isn't as fast as it should be, they may to return for visits every few months to see if their height catches up or if they should see a specialist to find possible causes.

I'm so tired all the time. I have to drag myself through classes and when I get home, I just lie on the couch and veg out. I have no energy. What's wrong with me?

You're not alone − a lot of teens feel tired. Your body is growing like crazy right now, so it's normal for you to feel rundown. Fortunately, there are ways to keep from feeling so fatigued. First, get plenty of sleep. If you can't get at least eight hours a night, try taking a short nap in the early afternoon.

An unbalanced diet can also zap your energy. Cut down on coffee and soda − they may perk you up for a little while, but you'll crash hard later. And don't skip meals! Food fuels your body and skipping a meal is like driving a car with an empty tank. Have a health snack after school to get your energy level back up. You may want to take a multivitamin every day because most teens don't manage to eat a balanced diet all the time. If you're still dragging despite all these healthy habit, talk to your doctor. You may need to be checked for anemia, thyroid problems or a viral infection.

I weigh ten pounds more than my sister and she is five years older than I am. Is something wrong with me?

There is nothing wrong with you − it's just that you're comparing apples and oranges. You can't compare your size with anyone else's, not even with your sister. Even within the same family, people can have very different eye and hair color or heights and weights.

Weight is only one factor to consider when wondering if you are a healthy size. If you compare equal amounts of muscle and fat, the muscle weighs much more. People who are taller have to weigh more too, because they have more bone and muscle. And people of the same height can have different healthy weights, depending on the size of their bone structure or muscle development.

At your next doctor visit, ask if your weight is appropriate for your height. Doctors calculate your body mass index to determine out if you are within the right range or if you should gain or lose weight to improve your health.

I sweat like crazy! I've tried all kinds of deodorants but nothing works. It's embarrassing! How can I stop it?

You may have a condition called hyperhidrosis, which means "too much sweating." In some people, the sweat glands in the hands, feet, groin, or armpits are overactive for no apparent reason. It can really affect your life, and worrying about it only makes the sweating worse.

So what can you do? First, tell your doctor about the problem. She may check your thyroid gland or ask if you're taking any medications that could be causing the sweating. She can also give you a prescription strength antiperspirant, which is applied overnight and used just once a week. There are other options for severe sweating, including Botox injections into the skin.

In the meantime, keep a container of antiperspirant in your bag and reapply it a few times during the day. This will help replace the antiperspirant that you sweat off. You can also try wearing cotton clothes which "breathes", unlike polyester, so your sweat has a chance to evaporate.

Lately, every time I eat (even a normal-size meal) I feel so sick that I think I'm going to throw up. What could be wrong?

Your question makes me wonder if you are afraid of being fat. Girls with eating disorders often restrict their diet so much that even a normal meal can seem way too much. This is due to their feelings about food and the way a normal amount of food feels in a stomach that has been kept empty.

Eating disorders can be tricky to recognize – family members and friends usually notice the signs before anyone else. Someone with an eating disorder may be aware of each and every thing they eat and know exactly how many calories or grams of fat it contains. They may exercise compulsively, like forcing themselves to do a certain number of sit-ups everyday or doing them after eating to use up the calories right away. People with eating disorders usually see too much fat when they look in the mirror, even if no one else sees it and they are actually underweight. They may also force themselves to throw up if they think they ate too much.

Eating disorders can spin out of control quickly and permanently damage health or even cause death. If any of the above description sounds like you, tell your doctor what is going on and get some help.

I hate peeing in public bathrooms, so at school I hold it in as long as I can. Is this safe?

No. Holding back on urinating can cause painful urinary tract infections. So when nature calls, start listening. When you wait too long, bacteria that have snuck into your bladder have plenty of time to multiply and cause problems. Skipping bathroom breaks on a regular basis can also cause your bladder to stretch out, leading to icky leaking problems in the future.

It is hard to catch any type of infection in a public bathroom, unless it's totally disgusting and you have open sores on your butt or thighs. If you're still wary of peeing in public, use seat covers or toilet paper to create a barrier between you and the toilet seat. Remember to wash your hands with plenty of soap before leaving the bathroom.

I have really bad mood swings. One minute I'm an angel and the next minute I'm sad and depressed. What is causing this and what can I do?

Mood swings are common during puberty and they usually get better over time. Your changing hormones levels during this time make it difficult to keep emotions under control.

Figure out how you best handle stress. Try exercising until you break a sweat several times a week, taking yoga classes, or learning relaxation exercises. Writing in a journal can help you express yourself without losing your cool in front of someone else.

If your mood swings are making you lose interest in school or friends or you have changes in your appetite or sleeping habits, you should see a doctor. Depression is dangerous if it becomes severe, which can happen without you much warning. If you've ever had thoughts about hurting yourself when you are feeling down, tell someone right away – a friend, a teacher, a relative, or your doctor.

Whenever I'm making out with my boyfriend, I get a weird tingling feeling, uh, down there. What's that about?

You didn't think kissing only involved lips, did you? Kissing and touching stimulates nerves in your skin and they send signals to your brain. With this information and the thoughts you've been thinking about your boyfriend, your brain releases chemicals that increase sexual arousal. This causes increased blood flow to your private parts, causing swelling of the labia minora and increased lubrication in the vagina. Your body does this in anticipation of possible sexual activity and it's all that blood flow that causes the tingling feeling. When you stop making out, the chemical signals from your brain stop and your private parts soon go back to feeling normal.

I have sweaty palms and every time my boyfriend and I hold hands, it seems to get worse. I'm really self-conscious about it. Is there anything I can do to stop this?

Don't sweat it! We all can get moist mitts when our nerves go into overdrive. Before you and your beau lock hands, give your palms a quick wipe on your clothes. Chances are if your hands are dry when your boyfriend first touches them, the sweat won't be as noticeable when it kicks up later. You could also try putting an underarm antiperspirant on your hands at bedtime and wash it off in the morning. Make sure it is an antiperspirant and not just a deodorant product, which won't help with sweating. It may be easier to apply if you use a liquid roller ball type than the solid stuff - it dries completely and won't get your bed sheets all messy.

If the sweating continues 24/7, you might have a condition called hyperhidrosis, which just means "excessive sweating." People with this condition also notice a lot of sweat on the soles of their feet and armpits. There are prescription strength antiperspirants that doctors can recommend to apply to sweaty spots once a week before going to sleep to help cut down on sweating. Tell your doctor if you take any medications on a regular basis because certain medications can make sweating problems worse. And remember to take a few deep breaths and try to chill out a little – being nervous makes the waterworks worse.

I have a weird problem: Sometimes I pee in my bed! It's so mortifying. What's wrong with me?

That is an embarrassing situation – but you're not the only teen with this problem. It sounds like you have a condition called enuresis (pronounced in-your-ee-sis), commonly known as bed-wetting. This happens more in guys, deep sleepers, and people who have a parent who had the problem. First, tell a doctor about it so they can rule out any medication conditions – like diabetes, a urine infection, or bladder weakness. Once you find out there's nothing medically wrong with you, you can start to tackle your problem.

Luckily, doctors and patients have found that changing some things your everyday life can help with this problem. Here are some tips: 1) Don't drink any liquids two hours before you go to bed. 2) Urinate right before you go to sleep. 3) Set an alarm clock for the middle of the night and get up to pee when it goes off. If these tricks don't work, your doctor might prescribe medication to help.

I went to a sleepover at my friend's house and everyone said I snored. I was so embarrassed. What can I do to stop this from happening again?

Don't lose sleep over it - snoring is common. It's just the sound of your nose and throat vibrating when you breathe deeply. For some people, it happens only when they're sick or have allergies. But a lot of people snore all the time and have not idea because they sleep in a room alone.

There are a few tricks you can try to quiet down snoring. Blow your nose before going to bed and if you have a cold or allergies, try taking a decongestant medication (ask your doctor or pharmacist to recommend one). Also, sleep on your side or your stomach. You're more likely to snore when you snooze on your back because your tongue drops back into your throat, blocking the airway. If all else fails, try using anti-snoring strips, which stick on the bridge of your nose and help keep the airways open. You should be resting easier in no time.

I get really bad stomachaches (like I have to go to the bathroom really bad) but it can take a few days before I'm able to go. What's wrong with me?

It sounds like you might be constipated. Constipation means that you have bowel movements less frequently than every one to two days or your bowel movements are small, hard, and possibly painful. There are often cramps and stomachaches that go along with constipation and you might even see a little blood on the toilet paper when you wipe. Many people with think that these symptoms are normal because they've had them so long, but the truth is they are just in constipation denial.

Most of the time, constipation can be managed with changes to your diet. Many people with constipation are dehydrated so drink plenty of water throughout the day to keep stool moist. Load up on fiber by eating fruits, vegetables, and whole grains and don't skip meals. If you can't get enough fiber in your diet, there are fiber supplements and shakes you can buy, but it's better to eat your fiber if you can. If these changes don't help, talk to your doctor before trying laxatives. While laxatives can be a quick fix in severe cases, if you use them regularly your body will become dependent on the laxatives to get your bowels moving and the constipation could get worse.

How do you know if some of the weird email rumors about certain products being dangerous are true or not?

Health and beauty products are used by more people than any type of prescription medication. (Who has *never* used shampoo or deodorant?) So really dangerous ingredients would be easily identified and those products would no longer be sold because there would be millions of people affected. However, there are some chemicals in commonly used products that have unknown safety records and may one day be recognized as unsafe. One option is stick to completely natural and organic products, but this will really limit your options for shampoo, skincare and makeup. A less extreme approach is to limit your exposure to these chemicals and alternate them with more natural products. It's similar to the chemicals in processed and non-organic foods – no one knows for sure how eating those over a lifetime will affect you when you are older.

Urban legends have been around for decades, but the internet has made it easy to spread rumors faster and to more people. My favorite way to check out these fake health alerts is by doing searches at snopes.com or urbanlegends.about.com - they have some of the most extensive lists of these panic provoking stories and the facts that prove they're wrong.

Can I catch anything from kissing my boyfriend?

Other than catching his attention, you can get a whole bunch of contagious things from kissing your boyfriend (or anyone, actually). Dry kissing is pretty safe, except for the chance of spreading cold sores, which are caused by a herpes virus infection spread by skin to skin contact. The sloppier the kiss, the bigger the chance of spreading an infection. Colds, flu, and strep throat are easy to catch through kissing. And why do you think mononucleosis - a viral infection that causes fever, sore throat and swollen lymph nodes – is nicknamed "the kissing disease?" Studies have also shown cavity-causing bacteria can be spread by kissing.

When it comes to sexually transmitted infections (STIs), the chance of spreading them by kissing is pretty slim. However, gonorrhea can hang out in the throats of people who had oral sex with someone who has a genital infection, causing a nasty sore throat. The HIV virus can be present in saliva, but in much lower concentrations than in blood or other body fluids so kissing is generally considered safe.

I think I have some sort of exercise disorder. I run 4 to 5 miles every day and then do about an hour of push ups and sit ups and weight lifting. I eat fine but I cannot stop exercising. It controls my life! Please tell me if I am exaggerating or if I really do need help and where to get it!

Sounds like you are truly obsessed with exercising. Any time someone feels a need to do something over and over, without being able to control or stop it, it's a problem that should not be ignored. You didn't say why you are doing all this exercise, which makes me wonder if you aren't sure yourself. Tell your doctor, teacher, school counselor, or parent and have them find you help. Many people put off getting help because they keep hoping these things will get better on their own, but they rarely do.

Out of control exercising can be part of Obsessive Compulsive Disorder (OCD), where people repeat activities (like counting or washing hands) and can't stop because they are afraid something bad will happen. Compulsive exercising can also be

64

due to an eating disorder, especially when exercising is done to burn up extra calories. Forcing yourself to exercise each time you ate too much or had an extra helping of dessert can be warning signs.

This is too embarrassing to ask my friends. For a few months now, I've been masturbating before I fall asleep at night. But I have a check up coming and I'm really scared that the doctor will be able to tell and be completely grossed out. Am I right?

Unless you've been touching yourself in a rough way that has caused cuts and scrapes down there, you doctor won't be able to tell that you've masturbated. While masturbation does cause changes in your body - an increased blood flow and sensitivity of the genitals – these changes are temporary.

Masturbation is a totally normal way of exploring your own body, so don't feel like your doctor would be grossed out. Many people do it, and you shouldn't be afraid to bring up the topic with your doctor if you have questions about masturbation. There really is nothing that you can tell your doctor that she hasn't heard before, so you should never be afraid to bring up health issues that concern you.

I constantly feel like I have to pee, and when I do, it hurts. Could this be serious?

Sounds like you might have a urinary tract infection, also now as a UTI or bladder infection. Besides the burning and a frequent need to urinate, some people even notice a little bit of blood in their urine. But don't worry, it's not as scary as it seems. Basically, a UTI develops when bacteria that's naturally living on the skin around your anus ends up in your urethra (the opening to the bladder). Most often this happens from having sex or wiping the wrong way after using the bathroom. Because of the way our bodies are designed, girls can get UTIs much easier than guys can.

Fortunately, UTIs are easy to get rid of with a short course of antibiotics, so make sure to see your doctor right away. Untreated UTIs can get worse and lead to kidney infections, which can be serious, are usually more painful with cramps and back pain, and sometimes require a stay in the hospital.

To prevent this from happening again, always wipe from front to back after going to the bathroom. Make sure to pee whenever you have the urge – don't wait until your bladder is about to burst. And, if you're having sex, urinate before and after you do the deed to help flush out a lot of the bacteria down there. You can also help prevent infections by drinking lots of water. Cranberry juice has been shown to help stop bacteria from sticking to the inside of the bladder, but avoid the ones with added sugar.

Someone told me wearing thong underwear causes hemorrhoids. Is this true?

Thongs may inspire some musicians to write songs, but they don't cause hemorrhoids, which are enlarged veins in the rectal area. Most people who have them don't even know it, unless they bleed or become painful, itchy and swollen. Hemorrhoids are common as people get older and usually are no big deal. You're more likely to get them if they run in your family or have problems with constipation, but rest assured knowing that you can don that thong without fear.

Keep this in mind: Too much of the thin thong crotch rubbing against your vaginal area *can* cause irritation of the skin down there. It's more likely to happen if those skinny undies are too tight or you wear them all the time. Switch to regular panties from time to time and skip thongs when you are exercise and sleeping. (It's actually a bad idea to wear *any* undies to bed.)

I'm on a low-fat diet to lose weight, but my social life revolves around hanging out at the diner with my friends! What can I order (besides a boring salad) that won't totally screw up my diet?

For starters, having fat in your diet is actually good for you, as long as it comes from healthy sources, such as olive oil and nuts - not fried foods. Your body makes hormones out of fat and if you don't get enough of it in your diet, your periods could get messed up. Brains and nerves are also made mostly of fat. So if you are going to limit some foods in your diet, try to cut out soda, foods with added sugar, and foods make from white flour – these things can cause weight gain and increase your risk of diabetes.

Forget the whole "diet" thing and focus on finding foods that are good for your body. Go for grilled chicken, turkey burgers, or fish and ask for veggies or a side salad instead of fries. If you are craving something sweet for dessert, try fresh fruits.

Help! I'm 14 and my body's maturing so much faster than all my friends' bodies – especially my boobs. Is there any kind of hormone or medicine I can take to slow it down?

While you're worrying whether you're growing too quickly, at least one of your friends is sure she's way behind on the puberty calendar. The fact is puberty is a process everyone goes through at their own pace. Some start early and breeze through at lightning speed while others don't finish developing until their mid twenties.

Doctors do prescribe hormone treatments in rare cases when puberty happens early in very young girls. But anything that would stop or slow down puberty at your age might permanently mess thing up and prevent you from ever fully maturing.

Unfortunately, it's hard to hide the fact that your body is changing, especially if you are the first of your friends to show it. Make sure to buy the right size bras and consider a wearing a sports bra during exercise for better support. Wearing shirts that are a little loose will also help ensure your chest isn't the first thing people notice about you.

My sister started to develop when she was 13. I'm already 14 and no signs yet. What could be wrong?

Everyone develops at their own pace, even within families and even twins! You and your sister may not have the same hair or eye color and may wind up being different heights, so why should this be any different?

However, just because you don't see any outward changes doesn't mean your body isn't already going through the first stages of puberty. Puberty starts before you see any changes in your body, so you might be on your way without even knowing it. In girls the first visible sign is usually enlargement of the nipples, followed by some pubic hair. Periods don't start until after breasts and pubic hair get really noticeable, and this can take anywhere from several months to a few years from when you first see any changes in your body.

Most of the time, developing later than your sisters or friends just means you are a bit of a late bloomer. Puberty can happen too slowly in some girls but it's not common. Any girl who hasn't had their period by age 16 should make an appointment with a doctor for an examination and maybe some blood tests to determine if there's a problem.

The guy I just started dating has a tongue ring. Do I have any reason to be worried about kissing him, like bacteria and other diseases? And is there anyway I could hurt him by smooching him too hard?

Well, your sweetie has a warm, moist, dark hole in his tongue – perfect for a spot to breed bacteria if a food particle gets stuck there. Occasionally, this can lead to infection – especially right after he's pierced, when the area around the hole hasn't healed. But unless you have a sore in your mouth, you probably won't catch anything from him – except maybe some scrapes on the inside of your mouth from his jewelry. Instead of worrying about hurting him, make sure you don't crack a one of your teeth or swallow his stud. Otherwise, you should be able to kiss without fear.

Sometimes after I've been making out with a guy, I get all of these red splotches on the skin around my neck and chest. Should I be worried?

Relax. The splotches are nothing to stress over. When you – or your guy – get excited from a major make-out session, your body reacts by pumping more blood to the face and upper chest area, sometimes causing redness. The flush usually fades about a half hour after you've stopped fooling around. If it doesn't – and our skin is also a little itchy – you could be sensitive to your date's cologne or aftershave. If he's got a mustache, goatee, or scruffy facial hair, that could be irritating your skin too, leaving you with a scratchy sunburn-like rash that's red and peels for a couple of days. One last possibility: If your boyfriend sucks on your skin when he kisses you, the suction could be causing a few capillaries to burst, leaving a blotch that looks like a reddish bruise. You may know them by their non-technical name – hickeys.

I'm 15 and I want to get my tongue pierced, but my mom won't let me. She says it will get infected. But isn't it totally safe?

Well, it's not *totally* safe. You run the risk of pain, infection and scarring. Bleeding is also a risk because there are lots of blood vessels under your tongue. Dentists also see tons of cracked teeth from metal jewelry.

In most states, parents need to give approval for body piercing done on anyone under 18 years old. So if your mom won't give in, you'll have to wait. Don't think about sneaking out someplace to have it done without permission or having a friend pierce you.

Always look for a clean piercing studio where the employees wear gloves and properly clean the skin they are going to pierce. Needles should be disposable and not reused, and tools need to be sterilized in an autoclave. If the place doesn't seem clean or if the piercer seems annoyed by your questions, walk out – no piece of jewelry is worth risking your health.

Tampon Troubles

I wore a tampon for a few hours, then I felt faint and had to sit down. After I took the tampon out, I was fine. Do I have Toxic Shock Syndrome?

Don't worry – what you experienced doesn't sound at all like Toxic Shock Syndrome (also called TSS). If you had that, you'd be *really* ill – and need emergency treatment. TSS symptoms include a high fever, a sunburn-like rash, peeling skin on the hands and feet, vomiting, diarrhea, and a sudden drop in blood pressure which makes you feel very dizzy (the "shock" part of TSS). Anyone with these symptoms needs to go to the hospital right away or else they could die.

Though it doesn't sound like you had TSS, since you use tampons, it's good to learn more about this serious illness. Toxic Shock Syndrome is *not* common – less than 20 of out 100,000 menstruating women get it. But when it happens, it can be deadly. TSS is cause by Staphylococcus aureus, a type of bacteria that normally lives on people's skin. If a large number of these bacteria grow in one area, they could make a dangerous poison that can get into the bloodstream through cuts in skin.

So how are tampons related to this rare illness? Bacteria love dark, moist, warm areas and tampons that are left in place for a long time give these bacteria the perfect place to multiply. And using a tampon when blood flow is light can result in tampon fibers attaching firmly to the vaginal wall, giving the bacteria a way to send their toxins into the body.

To decrease the risk of TSS, use less absorbent tampons, like junior/light flow/regular types so there's less chance of potential tampon irritation. You'll know if a tampon is too absorbent for you if it is hard to take out or if it leaves your vagina sore or dry. And use tampons during your period only – not before or afterwards. Also, don't leave a tampon in any longer than is recommended on the packages. Switching back and forth between tampons and pads is a good way to reduce tampon use and lessen the chances of TSS.

Why do I sometimes have trouble putting in a tampon? Sometimes it feels as if it didn't go in all the way and is really uncomfortable.

Using tampons can be tricky, especially when you first start trying to use them. To start, choose the smallest size you need (slim or junior ones for light days, regular for normal flow days, and super if you have heavy bleeding). Choosing the right tampon is important to reduce the chance of Toxic Shock Syndrome. The first time, try using a tampon on a day when your flow is a little heavy – it can make it easier to insert. Next, stand up and put one foot on the toilet seat. This makes the vaginal muscles relax and give you the best angle to put the tampon in. Hold the tampon in the middle of the applicator (there are sometimes ridges on the sides for an easier grip), insert it as deeply as you can and push the end of the applicator to release the tampon. If you're using a tampon without an applicator, keep pressure on the end of the tampon until you can't push it in any further. Remember to stay calm and relaxed. It may feel weird but you shouldn't be in any pain at ll. If you get nervous, try exhaling as you insert the tampon.

After the tampon is inserted and the applicator is removed, you shouldn't be able to feel the tampon at all. If you are walking around with any discomfort, you probably didn't put the tampon in deep enough. If this happens, take it out as soon as possible and try again.

When used correctly, tampons are safe, comfortable, and convenient. But they are just an option and some women chose to only use pads during their period. Another option is a menstrual cup, but that's much more complicated and a whole other discussion…

I got a scary email that said tampons contain asbestos. Is that true? Should I stop using them?

Tampons aren't dangerous, as long as you follow the directions on the box. They definitely *don't* contain asbestos. (In the US, they're regulated by the Food and Drug Administration, which means all their components have to be approved before they hit the shelf).

That rumor is just one of many internet hoaxes. The web makes it easy for rumors to spread; especially since well meaning friends can send these "warning" emails to everyone they know with the click of a mouse. But if we believed everything we read online, there would be mass hysteria over antiperspirants causing breast cancer, HIV-infected needles in movie theater seats and deadly spiders hiding in airport toilets – all myths.

You can check urbanlegends.about.com or snopes.com to check out most urban legends. Your best bet is to double check with your doctor anytime you come across info online that seems a little sketchy.

I've had my period for two months now. How long do I have to wait to use a tampon and is it hard to use?

There is no mandatory waiting time before you can use tampons. But, you need to be comfortable touching your body in order to insert tampons correctly. The very first time you try using one should be on a day when you have a heavy flow. This will make it slide in easier.

To insert a tampon, put one foot on the toilet seat to give yourself the best angle. Insert the applicator as deep as you can (remember to relax and try not to tense up) and then push the end in as far as it goes to release the tampon and remove the applicator. If done correctly, it shouldn't hurt and you shouldn't feel the tampon inside you. If you can feel it, it's not in deep enough – remove it and try again with a new one.

Once you start using tampons, be sure to pick ones with the right absorbency for your flow and don't leave them in for longer than eight hours. Alternating between tampons and pads is a good idea and will reduce your risk of Toxic Shock Syndrome, a rare but serious infection associated with tampon use. If you decide that tampons are not for you or you want to wait until you're a little older to try again, that's okay too.

I switched from pads to tampons, but I'm confused about how long you can leave them in. Is there such a thing as changing them too often?

As you probably know, leaving tampon in too long is a bad idea, because it gives the bacteria called Staphylococcus aureus a chance to breed inside of you. That can lead to a rare but serious condition called Toxic Shock Syndrome (TSS). But changing them too often can also be risky. If a tampon isn't soaked through when it's removed, it can scrape your vaginal walls, causing tiny open sores which could allow the bacteria to enter your bloodstream.

Generally, you can leave tampons in for up to eight hours, but changing them every 4 hours if they are soaked through is ideal. Alternating between tampons and pads will lower your risk of TSS. Just make sure to use the right absorbency for your flow. In other words, if your flow is light, opt for regular, slender, or junior tampons. Super absorbent tampons take longer to get fully saturated with blood, so they're more likely to be dry and rip the vaginal lining when removed. If you see white on the tampon or it's painful when removed, switch to a lower absorbency tampon. If you ever notice TSS symptoms (high fever, vomiting, diarrhea, severe dizziness, and a sunburn-like rash), remove your tampon and get medical help immediately.

I just got my period this month and I decided to try wearing tampons. But I couldn't get it in – it hurt too bad! Is there something wrong with me?

Tampons can be tricky at first, but with a little practice they're no big deal. To make insertion more comfortable, wait until the heaviest day of your cycle and use the smallest size tampon – either "junior" or "regular." Put one foot on the toilet seat and squat slightly. If you're nervous about using a tampon, your muscles may tighten and make it even more difficult. When you insert the tampon, relax the muscles around your vagina (as if you were going to urinate) so the tampon can slip in easier.

I pee often, so when I have my period I change my tampon every hour or two. But then I read that it's dangerous to change them so often. Can I just leave the tampon in there?

Urinating won't interfere with wearing a tampon – but it could slip out during a bowel movement from all that bearing down! There is no need to change your tampon every time you go to the bathroom. But you should use bathroom visits as opportunities to check to see if the tampon is becoming saturated and falling out in case you do need to change it at that time.

You're right – tampons shouldn't be changed *too* often. If it hasn't soaked up enough moisture, the tampon will cause small tears in the walls of your vagina, when it's pulled out. This can increase the risk of Toxic Shock Syndrome, a rare but dangerous bacterial infection.

Can you swim with a tampon in? My friend does that but I always thought that during your period you were not supposed to do any sports, so swimming should be a double no-no on your period, right?

In the olden days, people thought that women needed to avoid all forms of exercise during their period because it was dangerous. But we now know that's not true and you can do almost any sports during your period that you do the rest of the month. And swimming is no exception - thanks to tampons.

Tampons will absorb water from a bath or pool and may not last as long inside you as they would if you were not in water. So, it's a good idea to put a new tampon in right before getting into the pool and change it as soon as you are done swimming. You may want to consider using tampons that are more absorbent in the pool than you usually use.

I hate wearing pads to bed because they always leak during the night. Is it okay to wear tampons overnight?

Tampons can lead to TSS (toxic shock syndrome) if you use ones that are too absorbent for your amount of flow or if you leave them in too long. Tampons can be worn safely for up to 8 hours at a time, no matter what time of day you put them in. So, if you're planning to sleep 8 hours or less, you can wear a tampon overnight but don't forget to remove it in the morning. But if you know that you're planning to sleep in all day, you're better off using a pad -- try extra-long "overnight pad" or ones with wing-like side coverage to help prevent leakage.

I already have my period, and I'm only 12! Am I too young to wear a tampon?

It sounds like you've started your period before several of your friends, but you're not really an early bloomer compared with the rest of the country. It's normal for periods to start as early as age 8 or as late as age 16.

The decision about when to start using tampons is a personal one which depends more on when you feel comfortable touching yourself in order to use them, rather than how old you are. And no one is *required* to use tampons – some women choose to stick with pads their whole lives.

If you want to experiment with tampons, wait until your next period and pick a day with heavier flow. Choose the smallest tampons with an applicator you can find – they're usually called "junior". Read the instructions in the package carefully – most have detailed instructions and diagrams to show you how to insert a tampon. The package inserts also have important information about toxic shock syndrome (TSS), a dangerous infection associated with tampon use. The risk of TSS with tampons is low if you only wear tampons when you have your period, don't take them out soon after putting them in, or don't wear them for more than 8 hours at a time.

Is it possible to "lose" a tampon?

Only if it drops out of your hand and you can't see where it rolled away to… But seriously, this is a very common question because many women aren't familiar with their own anatomy. The vaginal canal is pretty much a dead end, with the exception that the tiny opening in the cervix leads into the uterus, with two small openings through the fallopian tubes to the ovaries and lower abdomen. Something the size of a tampon can't go anywhere else inside your body.

If you put a tampon in and can't find it there are a few possible explanations: 1) it fell out without you knowing it - which can happen if you're constipated or pushing hard when having a bowel movement, 2) you thought you used a tampon but didn't, or took it out and forgot, or 3) the string broke and you can't reach it (but you'd probably know if the string wasn't there when you put it in). Doctors sometimes have to retrieve tampons that lost their strings or that have been left in too long and become stuck.

PMS Distress

When I have PMS, I turn into a real bitch! All my friends get mad at me. Is there any way I can calm down?

As if cramps weren't bad enough, lots of girls have to deal with crazy mood swings during their periods. Because the symptoms of premenstrual syndrome (PMS) are different in everyone, there aren't any guaranteed tricks for beating the monthly blues. But there are a few suggestions that are worth trying.

Exercising a few times a week is good for your body and can help relieve some of the stress that builds up and gets out of control before your periods. If you can't bear the thought of working out, try some relaxation exercises, like medication or yoga. These can also help you chill out and control your emotional outbursts.

When you know you're about to get your period, don't forget to watch your diet. Not getting enough vitamins and minerals can make PMS worse. Taking a multivitamin and getting plenty of calcium and magnesium in your diet may make you feel a little more balanced – and eating healthy is always a good idea. Finally, have a heart-to-heart with your friends and let them know that you can't always control your mood when you're dealing with PMS. If they know not to take your mood swings personally, you can avoid misunderstandings in the future.

I get really bloated, crampy, and moody before my period. I take over the counter pills and other pain killers for my period symptoms, but nothing seems to work. Is there anything else I can to do to beat my PMS hell?

PMS symptoms are different for everyone. But there are some things you can try. Avoid salty foods during the week before your period to cut down on the water retention. If over-the-counter pain relievers don't work well enough, ask your doctor to prescribe you a stronger version. And if the cramps persist, you might consider taking birth control pills – even if you've never had sex – to regulate your period and help with the cramps.

Moodiness is often the hardest PMS symptoms to treat. Some women find doing regular exercise, taking calcium and magnesium supplements, or eating more carbohydrates during your period helps. Sometimes treating the bloating and cramps can make you less crabby too.

Battle PMS pain the same way as you would period cramps. Use a heating pad or use a medication like ibuprofen or naproxen. Regular exercise can also help relieve stress and control the bloating that happens during that time of month.

Doctors use anti-depressant medications for PMS mood swings, but it's only used in severe cases and it has to be taken every day or for two weeks before each period for it to help.

I get PMS really bad. I become depressed and moody – I even cry a lot. What can I do?

When hormones go wild the week before your period, it can be a real body bummer – physically and emotionally. Premenstrual Syndrome (PMS) usually refers to the physical symptoms – bloating and cramping – and Premenstrual Dysphoric Disorder (PMDD) is a new term for the emotional and psychological symptoms. Most women get a little crabby and emotional that time of the month. The good news is that when your period starts each month, the symptoms of usually disappear. But until they do, here are tips for making PMDD more bearable.

Whether you get weepy for no reason or suffer from mood swings, cutting back on caffeine (coffee tea, cola) might help you stay mellow. Since caffeine makes a person more wired and agitated anyway, it makes sense that cutting it out might help. Avoiding sugary and fried foods – the kind of stuff most women crave during their periods – can also help. Many women find that boosting their calcium and magnesium intake also helps with moodiness. In fact there are several studies that show calcium helps with both the physical and emotional symptoms women experience before their periods– make sure you get at least 1000 mg of calcium a day from calcium-rich foods. If your symptoms start to get in the way of school and your social life, see a doctor. Antidepressant medications are used for treating PMDD, but they need to be taken for the two weeks before each period or everyday and we don't know if they continue to work if taken for more than 6 months.

Is there anything you can take for PMS mood swings? I can't function at all when I get my period. Should I ask my doctor about starting anti-depression medication?

PMS can be a real pain and as many as 70 percent of women suffer from it. But before you turn to prescription medication, there are some things you can try on your own to feel better. Strive to get regular exercise and avoid stressful situations. Some women find magnesium, calcium and B vitamin supplements help.

If your symptoms persist, talk to your doctor about medication. Birth control pills often relieve physical and emotional symptoms by controlling hormone levels. Prescription anti-depressant medications like fluoxetine and paroxetine help some women but it only lessens the emotional symptoms and they haven't been studied in teenagers. Paroxetine has been approved in the US for treating PMDD (Premenstrual dysphoric disorder), the emotional symptoms from PMS, but it needs to be taken every day or for two weeks before each period. Although medicine may be necessary, changing your lifestyle a bit may be enough to make PMS tolerable.

Need to Know: Normal or Not?

Sometimes when I have my period, the blood is dark and clumpy. Is there something wrong with me?

Dark, clumpy blood isn't unusual or a sign that anything is wrong. When you menstruate, you bleed because the lining of your uterus is being shed. The lining grows thicker during your cycle and when there's no pregnancy at the end of cycle, the lining falls out over several days. The lining can come off in small or large pieces, which is probably what you're noticing. Menstrual blood sticks to the larger pieces and they can look extra clumpy.

Blood that's been in the vagina for a while also tends to look dark and turn into clots – so don't freak out about that either. That's why women are more likely to see blood clots in the mornings during their periods. Just remember what your period looks like every month, so if you notice something really unusual you can see a doctor to make sure everything is okay. Everyone's cycle is different, so try to be aware of what's normal for you and what's not.

Help! I'm 14 and haven't gotten my period yet. All of my friends have theirs. What's wrong with me?

Absolutely nothing is wrong with you. Generally, menstruation begins between the ages of 9 and 16. Why the huge span? Every girl's body develops at its own pace, so you may not yet be making enough of the hormones you need to jump start puberty until months – or even a couple of years – after your friends do. And after these hormones are released, they can take a while to work together properly for you to get monthly periods. So if you think you're the only girl on the planet who hasn't started her period, rest assured you have lots of company. And remember: this doesn't mean you haven't started becoming a woman yet. Menstruation is one of the last things to happen during puberty. Other changes, like pubic hair and breast development, come long before your first period.

If there's no sign of your period by age 16, tell your doctor who can make sure your hormones are all in check. Meanwhile, realize your friends aren't enjoying their periods and most wish they were still waiting for their periods to start like you are.

Sometimes during my period, the blood on my tampon looks really brown. Other times it looks bright red. What's up with that?

Even though blood might look bright red when it first comes out of you, it starts to darken as soon as it's exposed to air. (Just think of the last time you scraped your knee and were left with a brownish scab the next day.) That means the longer you leave your tampon in, the more time your blood will have to darken.

The end where the string is attached may look darkest, since it's constantly exposed to outside air. But how does the rest of your tampon darken when it's inside you? Believe it or not, a teeny bit of air is always inside the vagina. That's why you've probably noticed that your blood is brownest on your lightest days – when it's trickling out more slowly. Not only is this when your flow takes longest to leave your body, but since you also don't need to change your tampons as often the blood can end up sitting in your vagina for a while. Aren't you glad you asked?

I'm 15 and I masturbate kind often. Is that why I haven't gotten my period yet?

Masturbation won't speed up or slow down puberty. It has no long-term side effects and it isn't bad for you health unless you spend *so* much time doing it that you stop hanging out with friends of doing other activities.

Some girls are close to16 years old before they get their first period. Don't worry if all of your friends have their periods already – consider yourself lucky that you are spared several more months without cramps and PMS!

This is kind of gross, but whenever I have my period, I get diarrhea. Why does that happen?

When you shed the lining of your uterus during your period, your body releases chemicals called prostaglandins. Not only do they cause cramps but, they also increase the movement of your intestines, which can cause diarrhea. Many women notice looser stools right before their period. It's annoying but, like cramps, you usually only have to deal with it the first day or two of your cycle. You can try a non-prescription medication for diarrhea. Medications like ibuprofen and naproxen may help with both the diarrhea and the cramps. Bottom line: your period really can be a pain in the ass in more ways than one!

I hate having periods and can't handle the sight of blood anywhere, especially from my own body. The sight of blood makes me anxious, nauseated and want to faint! For a week each month I'm miserable. Is there was a way to make my periods go away until I get older and am ready to have babies?

Your wish is a common one among young girls with their periods. Interestingly, there are ways of making periods much less frequent, with some forms of birth control. Women who use the birth control injection (also known as depot medroxyprogesterone acetate) often have no menstrual cycles after the first couple of shots, but they might have light spotting every day for the first three months. There are also extended birth control pill formulations, with three months of hormone pills in each pack that makes periods come every 3 months – or just 4 periods a year.

Talk to your doctor about options for managing your period and talk to your parent to see if they are okay with you taking medications. Hormonal forms of birth control have side effects, so if you are using them for more convenient cycles and not preventing pregnancy, you need to determine if the risks are worth the benefits.

Sometimes I get this really weird smell down there when I'm having my period. I'm a virgin, so it doesn't have anything to do with sex. Can other people smell it? What is wrong with me?

Relax – there's probably nothing wrong with you. Vaginal odor is common and, luckily, it's not usually something other people notice. Menstrual fluid doesn't normally smell until it comes in contact with the bacteria in the air and on your skin. So when you bleed into a pad, it can start to get funky. Here are some non-stinky solutions: Change pads more often, wear cotton underwear, and gently wash the vaginal area with a mild soap. Also, skip scented pads and tampon and avoid deodorant sprays that can irritate the skin and make problems worse. Some women also find there is less odor when they use tampons, so that might be something to consider. If you notice a funky smell *after* your period ends, it could be bacterial vaginosis, a treatable imbalance in the vagina's bacteria that can be checked out by your doctor.

Okay, I *cannot* ask any of my friends about this. I masturbate kind of often, and I still haven't gotten my period. Can masturbating screw up your period?

Masturbation has no long-term side effects and isn't bad for your health unless you spend so much time doing it that you aren't spending time with friends and doing other activities. Babies discover early on that it feels good to touch themselves down there – check out where their hands automatically go during diaper changes! Masturbating also won't speed up or slow down puberty and development.

It can be tough if all of your friends have a head start on puberty and you're straggling behind a bit. Normally, periods usually start before age 16. If you still have no period after that age, ask your doctor to check you out to make sure that you're just a late bloomer and that there isn't a hormonal reason for not having periods yet.

Irritatingly Irregular Cycles

Sometimes I have this brownish-red discharge the week after my period. Is it my period coming back? What's wrong with me?

Some periods start or end with spotting – the light menstrual flow that looks like a brownish discharge. It happens more often in women with short periods (only a few days of bleeding) and is nothing to worry about. Also, periods can do strange things in beginning, so your periods may not be like this forever if you had your first period less than two years ago.

Spotting between periods can also happen with birth control pills. If it continues, your doctor can usually fix things by switching you to a different pill. The birth control injection can cause frequent spotting at first, but it usually stops after the second dose and then periods may come only once every 3 months. If you never had any spotting before, it could be a sign of a sexually transmitted disease or pregnancy and should be checked out by a doctor

My periods are totally unpredictable. Sometimes my period lasts only two days and other times it lasts for over a week. I've never had sex, so I'm not worried about being pregnant, but it drives me crazy. This can't be normal!

Don't stress – it *is* normal. Your period can be very weird the first couple of years – it might skip a month or come too often. But even after the first few years, it's common to have irregularities. First of all, not everyone has a 28-day cycle. In fact, some women's cycles are never totally normal. And other factors can make your periods wacky, like stress, a poor diet, and excessive exercise. But it's still a good idea to keep track of your periods and then go see a doctor.

Start by marking the first day of your period on a calendar and, after a few months, count the days between the marks. Also, mark the days you bleed and note if it is heavy or light. This will help your doctor figure out what's going on. If your periods are still a mess, the doctor might prescribe birth control pills to help regulate your cycles.

I'm not sexually active, but sometimes I'll go several months without getting my period. Do I have a problem?

Skipping periods no w and then isn't a problem. In fact, most women miss a month or two now and then because of stress, illness, or a rapid change in weight. It's also common for periods to be irregular for the first few years you have them. So if you just started having periods if you skip once in a while, there's probably nothing wrong. But some menstrual periods are never regular and some get more spaced out as time goes on, both of which suggest there could be a problem. A common cause of having infrequent periods is a hormonal imbalance called Polycystic Ovarian Syndrome (PCOS), where the ovaries develop lots of little, painless, and fluid-filled pockets. Lots of women have this problem, although some women don't even realize it. Other symptoms of PCOS include acne, more facial and body hair, and weight gain.

So if your periods are very irregular, you should see a doctor who can tell you what is going on after ordering some blood tests to check your hormone levels. PCOS is usually treated with birth control pills to regular period cycles or with a medication called metformin, which is usually used to treat diabetes (because PCOS is also associated with a problem with insulin, the hormone that regulates blood sugar levels).

I'm not sexually active but sometimes I go for months without getting my period. I'm 15 – do I have a problem?

Probably not. The first two years after your period starts can be unpredictable. I t might skip months, show up when you least expect it, or be super heavy or ultra light. But don't worry – after two years you should settle into what will be a normal cycle for you. (A "normal" cycle can be anywhere from 21-40 days, from the first day of one period to the first day of the next).

So why else might you be having period-free periods? Of course, if you were having sex, there would be the possibility you could be pregnant. Some pregnant women have intermittent bleeding that can trick them into thinking that they aren't pregnant. Even if you're not having sex, you cycle might stop if you go through a stressful situation (like a death in the family or major surgery) or if you lose too much weight and body fat (from sports training, dieting or being sick). In these cases, your body's survival instincts kick in and focus all your energy on healing or staying alive instead of reproduction. Periods usually get back to normal once the stress passes or weight returns to normal.

Usually the toughest cycle-stoppers to identify are thyroid problems or hormone imbalances, because the other symptoms associated with them are subtle. In general, a good rule of thumb is if you skip more than two periods, you should see a doctor. You might need your thyroid and hormone levels checked and, if you've had sex, be sure to ask for a pregnancy test.

I'm 14 and sometimes I have this brownish-red discharge the week after my period. Is it my period coming back? What's wrong with me?

Periods can be strange – especially in the first two years. Sounds like you just have "spotting," a light menstrual flow that can look kind of brownish. Some periods start or end with spotting – especially if your period is super light or only lasts a few days. The blood has turned brown because it's been exposed to air. (It's brighter red when your period is heavier and flowing at a faster rate.)

To make it a little more tolerable – and to keep your underwear stain-free – wear a thin panty-liner for the week after your period or until it's completely finished. If this spotting continues the whole time between your periods, see your doctor. It could be a sign of infection, pregnancy, or side effects from birth control pills. It could also lead to anemia from loss of too much blood.

I am 14 and just got my first period 2 months ago, but it hasn't stopped for a single day since it started. The bleeding is so heavy that I sometimes need to change my pad every couple of hours. I heard that periods are usually irregular at first but I can't handle this!

It is definitely NOT normal for periods to last more than a week, especially if the bleeding is heavy much of that time. You need to see a doctor immediately to make sure that you haven't lost a dangerous amount of blood and need a blood transfusion to return your levels to normal.

Some girls are unable to clot their blood well, because they don't make some of the critical factors our bodies use to stop bleeding. Many of these girls have no idea they have this problem until their first period (because they never had a major cut or a car accident when it would have been discovered earlier). Blood tests can determine if this is your problem and what treatment is needed. Other causes for heavy bleeding include hormonal imbalances, which are often treated with birth control pills for several months to regulate cycles.

I just started my period a few months ago, but I get it every two weeks! It's so annoying. How often am I supposed to get it? Do I have to deal with this forever? I feel like it's that time of the month *all the time*!

A few lucky girls start off with regular monthly cycles from the start, but most wind up with periods that are too close together or too spaced out at first. It can take up to a year for your cycles to become regular after they start. And for cycles that don't settle into a regular pattern after a year, birth control pills are often used to keep them on track.

With periods that happen every 2-3 weeks is that you could be losing more blood than if you had a period every month. Taking a multivitamin with iron each day isn't a bad idea. If you have more than 7 days of bleeding during your periods, have to change tampons or pads several times a day because they're soaked, feel tired or dizzy more than usual, or look paler than normal – you should have a doctor check you out for anemia (low levels of red blood cells).

I know that it's normal to have irregular periods at my age, but I used to be super regular and I haven't had a period in six months. Could there be something wrong?

The first thing to ask yourself is "Could I be pregnant?" If you've had sex within the past year, get tested now – even if you used birth control. If you're not pregnant, a couple of other things could be going on and you should see a doctor to help figure it out what is making your periods go missing.

During the first couple of years of menstruation, your body has to get used to a ton of new hormones. Since it takes a while for all of them to get in sync, even a regular cycle and get tripped up sometimes from minor stuff like stress, or a change in sleep patterns.

A serious illness or rapid weight loss can interfere with your period and could even make you completely stop menstruating for a long period of time. Other causes of irregular menses include Polycystic Ovarian Syndrome (PCOS), which is caused by a hormonal imbalance and is usually associated with worsening acne and increased body hair.

I got my period 5 months ago and every month it seems to come later and later in the month? Is this serious?

You may count the months going by with a calendar, but your body sees time differently. Periods average a 28 day cycle (but can be a week more or less and still normal) and the cycles are counted from the first day of one cycle to the first day of the next - no matter how many days you bleed. Because February is the only month that is 28 days long, as time goes by you'll find your periods <u>earlier</u> in the following month and you may get two periods in the same month if the first one starts on the first few days of the month and the second one comes at the end of the month.

The first two years of having your period can be kind of weird, with periods that skip months or are closer together than normal. This is because your body is adjusting to the hormonal changes and hasn't yet gotten into the groove of a regular cycle. A good way to try to predict your periods is marking them out on a calendar and seeing if you can't predict them after a few months. This will hopefully help you avoid any unpleasant surprises. Periods where bleeding lasts more than 7 days or periods are coming closer than 3 weeks apart should be checked out by a doctor.

I just got my period for the first time. But I've heard that your period can be totally irregular the first year, and I'm so scared that I'm going to get "surprised" one day at school. Is there any way to know when you're about to get your period?

Unfortunately, it's normal for menstrual cycles to be irregular for the first two years after they start. Usually, these irregular cycles skip a month or more between periods but many girls start having monthly cycles from the beginning. But even when cycles are very regular, periods may come a day or two earlier or later than expected.

While there is no magic sign that your period is about to begin, there are a few clues you can use to figure out when you really need to be carrying a supply of tampons or pads with you. Breasts tend to get sore before a period starts, because the higher hormone levels affect breast tissue and cause fluid retention. If you notice that you get moodier than normal before your periods you may be able to guess when a period is about to start. Some women also have lower abdominal cramping that starts before a period. Women often report that they feel that they feel like they have to urinate right around the time their periods start each month. Pay attention the next time your period starts – you may be able to use some of these hints to predict your periods.

Until your cycles get regular, it can't hurt to wear a pantyliner on days when you think your period might come – based on your calendar or some of your body's signals which hint that your period may be around the corner. You may also want to carry a tampon or pad (and maybe an extra pair of underwear) in your school bag to help minimize the mess of an unexpected period.

I'm 15 and used to have really light, easy periods, but lately my flow has been getting a lot heavier. I've also been getting really bad cramps. Is this supposed to happen or should I worry?

It takes a couple of years after your first period for your cycle to even out and find its groove, so it's possible that the heavier, longer periods you've been having lately are normal for you. Normal periods last between two and eight days and come 21 to 40 days apart – in other words, there's a huge range from one girl to the next. Weight loss, birth control pills, and stressing about whether your cycle is normal can also shake things up.

Most girls think they bleed more than they actually do, but if you're not sure, here's a good rule of thumb: You're probably not bleeding too much if you use one pad at a time or don't soak through super-sized tampons or pads every 2 to 3 hours. If you are bleeding that much, tell your doctor. As for your cramps, heating pads and an over-the-counter anti-inflammatory medication, like ibuprofen or naproxen, should help with the pain. If not, ask your doctor about prescription medications for period cramps.

Cramps Cramping Your Style?

Most of my friends get crampy during their periods, but my pain actually starts *before* my period. Is this normal?

Totally normal. This is one of those odd PMS facts. During the week before a period, some of us feel moody, some feel crampy, some feel both moody and crampy, and some feel nothing at all. And despite what many people (especially guys) PMS is not all in your head. PMS symptoms, which include bloating and emotional highs and lows, are all due to the changes in your hormone levels that happen as your uterus prepares to shed its lining. Of course, that shedding process is what causes the cramps you feel during your period. But since the uterus is actually one big muscle, the pain you get *before* your period may feel more like a dull muscle ache, mainly caused by the blood vessels in the lining starting to detach.

My cramps hurt so much during my period. I take ibuprofen, but what else can I do to ease the pain?

Having cramps can be a bummer. Luckily, there are some things you can do to lessen the pain. You just need to experiment to see what works best for you. Over-the-counter drugs containing ibuprofen are most effective if you take them right when your period or cramps start. These medications should help to lessen the muscle cramps because of their anti-inflammatory action. (Acetaminophen-containing medications aren't as effective in treating cramps because they don't treat inflammation and swelling.) If ibuprofen doesn't work for you or you need to take it every 4 to 6 hours, you may want to try over-the-counter naproxen, which is stronger and lasts longer. All of these medications should be taken with food so they don't upset your stomach. You can also try putting a heating pad or hot water bottle on your stomach to help relax the muscles. Increasing the amount of calcium-rich foods you eat right before your period – things like milk, cheese and other dairy foods – might also help lessen the pain.

If none of these remedies help and your cramps are keeping you from doing to school or doing any of your normal activities, you should see a doctor who might prescribe birth control pills to ease the pain. The Pill helps prevent cramps from starting by blocking ovulation and, in many cases, period cramps may go away completely while they are taken.

I get killer cramps – like, I can barely stand up straight. Is something wrong? And is there anything I can do to relieve them?

Cramps suck but there's no reason to suffer every month. The quickest way to fight cramps is with an over-the-counter painkiller, like ibuprofen or naproxen. Take it as soon as you feel the first twinge of cramping – the longer you wait, the less likely it is that *anything* will help. For some girls, stretching or exercising can help relieve cramps, but if you can't bear to move, lie down and apply a heating pad to your belly (just don't fall asleep with it because you could get burned).

If your cramps are too tough for these tricks, talk to your doctor – especially if you have to miss school often because of period pain. She may be able to prescribe a stronger painkiller or she may recommend birth control pills to regulate your cycle and make your period less painful. Even if you haven't had sex yet, birth control pills are commonly used to treat period problems, including severe cramps, heavy bleeding, and irregular cycles.

Going to a Gynecologist

What happens at the gynecologist?

Visiting a gynecologist is weird or scary, but it shouldn't hurt. You should tell the doctor or nurse that it's your first time, so they can explain things to you before the exam begins. Schedule your appointment for a time when you won't be on your period and don't have sex or put anything in your vagina for two days ahead of time.

The doctor will ask you about your menstrual cycle, if you've ever had sex, and what you have used for birth control. Don't be embarrassed – doctors ask everyone the same questions and being honest with your answers will make sure you get the best medical care. Your examination may include a breast exam (depending on your age) and a vaginal exam. If you've never had sex, the vaginal exam will be brief.

If you've had sex, you'll need to have a complete exam. You will put your feet in foot rests, lie back, and scoot your butt to the end of the exam table. The outside of the vagina will be examined to make sure there you're healthy. Then, to examine your cervix, a metal or plastic instrument called a speculum is inserted into the vagina. Swabs are used to test for gonorrhea and Chlamydia. If you're over 21 years old, a Pap smear is done to check for abnormal cells on the cervix. The speculum is removed and the size and shape of your ovaries are checked, by the doctor placing two fingers inside the vagina with another hand pressing on your lower belly. It sounds like a lot, but the whole exam takes only about ten minutes. You may also be sent to a lab for blood tests for syphilis and HIV. One of the best ways to have a less stressful exam is to try to relax during the whole thing. Take deep breaths, let your legs feel heavy, and pick a point on the ceiling to stare at.

This is too embarrassing to ask my friends. For a few months now, I've been masturbating before I fall asleep at night. But I have check up coming up at the doctor's office, and I'm really scared that the doctor will be able to tell and she'll be completely grossed out. Am I right?

Unless you've been touching yourself in a rough way that has caused cuts or scrapes down there, your doctor won't be able to tell that you've masturbated. While masturbation does cause changes in your body – such as increased blood flow and sensitivity of the genitals – these changes are temporary.

Masturbation is a totally normal way of exploring your own body, so don't feel like your doctor would be grossed out. Most people do it, and you shouldn't be afraid to bring up the topic with your doctor if you have questions about masturbation. There's nothing you can tell your doctor that she hasn't heard before, so you should never be afraid to bring up health issues that concern you.

I made an appointment to see the gynecologist, but I've never been before. What should I expect?

It's normal to be a little nervous the first time. But don't worry – it might be weird, but it shouldn't hurt. It helps to tell the doctor or nurse this is your first time so they can talk to you about what to expect before you have to get undressed.

Here's what will happen: First the doctor will ask you about your menstrual cycle, if you're sexually active, and if you are, what you're using for birth control. Next, she'll examine you, which may include a breast exam and a vaginal exam (and that's the part most girls feel funny about): You put your feet in the foot rests at the end of the exam table, lie back, and scoot your butt to the end. She'll look at the outside of the vagina to make sure you're healthy. Then, she may insert a metal or plastic speculum (an instrument that helps the doctor see your cervix) inside your vagina. She may also do tests with a swab for gonorrhea and Chlamydia, and may do a Pap smear, which is a test that detects abnormal cells on the cervix. Afterwards, she may check the size and shape of your ovaries and uterus by placing two fingers inside the vagina and using her other hand to press on your lower belly. It sounds like a lot but the whole thing lasts only about 10 minutes. You may also be sent to get blood tests for infections like HIV and syphilis.

I'm sexually active, and my boyfriend and I use condoms. I want to go on birth control, too, to be even safer. But my friend says the only way to get birth control is to go to the gyro. I'm so grossed out by the idea of someone looking

around down there. Is there any other way to get birth control pills?

In the US, the only way to get birth control pills is to have a doctor, nurse practitioner, or physician assistant write you a prescription. This is to make sure that you understand the increased risks of some health problems – blood clots in legs, gallbladder stones and possibly a higher risk of breast cancer – before you start taking birth control pills. (Don't worry – there are lots of potential benefits too – like not getting pregnant and a lower risk of ovarian cancer). There are also lots of options to pills these days too – injections, patches that you wear for a week at a time, rings that you wear inside your vagina for three weeks. Your healthcare provider can tell you about them so that you can find a method that's right for you.

Once you've had sex or after age 21, it's important to have regular gynecological exams to make sure that you don't have any hidden sexual health problems. An exam isn't absolutely necessary before starting pills, but most doctors know that you're less likely to come back for an exam at another time if you don't have one done at your first visit. So, schedule your appointment for a time when you don't think you'll be on your period so you can get everything taken care of at one visit.

I started having sex recently and want to visit a gyno. But when I asked my mom she got suspicious! How can I convince her to let me without filling her in on my sex life?

You'd have to be pretty sneaky to get to the gynecologist without your mom finding out, so remind her that going to a gynecologist is a healthy choice, even when you're *not* having sex, Tell her that you want to be responsible about your health – regular gynecological visits can help detect early forms of cancer and your doctor can teach you how to do a breast self-exam.

If your mom still freaks out at the idea or if you absolutely *can't* handle having your parents find out you went for a checkup, call a Planned Parenthood office. They usually charge a low fee for a gynecologic exam and are generally friendly to younger patients. All visits for reproductive health issues should be confidential – so even if your parents ask, your doctor can't tell them if you're sexually active, pregnant, or have an STI (sexually transmitted infection) unless the situation is life threatening. These laws were made to ensure that you can take care of your sexual health, even if your parents don't know you're having sex.

I have to go to the gynecologist and I'm freaking out about getting a Pap smear! I'm totally embarrassed. Why do I need one?

The good news is that the recommendation for Pap smears was recently changed. Instead of starting to get them yearly, starting when you first have sex, Pap smears are now only done starting at age 21. This change was made because abnormal cells on the cervix are often found from the human papillomavirus (HPV) but in young women most of the time they became normal again and rarely turn into cancer cells. But once you start having sex, you should be tested for sexually transmitted infections at least once a year.

It may seem weird to have you doctor getting so up close and personal with you, but no need to get embarrassed – this is what she does for a living! During a Pap smear, the doctor collects cells from the cervix (the opening to the uterus) and sends them out for testing for cancerous or other abnormal cells. Some women feel minor cramping, but it's pretty painless. Testing for STIs is usually done as well. The doctor also does an internal exam to make sure the size and shape of your uterus and ovaries are normal. The whole visit is usually over in 15 minutes, so it's really no big deal.

Virgin Verifications

Can a gynecologist tell if you're sexually active just by examining you?

There is no definite way for a doctor to tell if you've ever had sex. People used to think that a doctor could tell if you were a virgin by seeing if your hymen – the thin rim of skin around the opening of the vagina, - was intact, but that's a myth. They hymen can tear before a woman ever has sex (common culprits include strenuous exercise and riding a bicycle). It's also possible that a stretchy hymen won't ever tear, even after someone has sex many times. Some women are even born with almost no hymen at all. Despite all this, the myth of doctors being able to do a "sex check" is still around but it just isn't true.

You should be prepared for your doctor to ask you if you've ever had sex and it's important that you tell the truth. Don't worry that they will judge you - believe me, they've heard this all before! They need to know so you can be checked for possible infections and be given birth control information. Don't stress about your doctor telling your parents about your sexual status – most states in the US prohibit doctors from telling anyone, even your parents, about your sexual history unless you are in danger. You may have many questions about sexuality or birth control- write them down in advance so you don't forget to ask them while you're in the office.

My boyfriend and I had sex for the first time, but we were both really nervous and we stopped halfway through. So, am I still a virgin?

Different people have their own concepts about virginity, but the most commonly accepted definition is that if a penis goes into a vagina, even a little, virginity is lost. It's kind of like football – it doesn't matter how far you run past the goal line, it's just that you cross it.

So what does this mean for you? Doctors use the same definition when asking patients if they've ever had sex, because even this low-level of sexual activity can put you at risk for STIs and pregnancy - meaning that you should get checked out like a sexually active woman.

My boyfriend and I were alone at his house yesterday, so we, um, took advantage of the situation. While we were making out, he put his finger inside me – and I started bleeding! Does this mean I'm not a virgin anymore?

It's tough to define virginity, but most people agree that it means someone who hasn't had sexual intercourse. According to that definition, genital touching doesn't count. So what happened during your hot-and-heavy makeout session? Your boyfriend touched your hymen, the thin ring of skin around the opening to your vagina. When the hymen is stretched or ripped, during sex or when something is inserted in the vagina, it may start to bleed a little.

People used to believe that as soon as your hymen was broken, you lost your virginity. But today, we know that's not true – you can break your hymen by using tampons, playing sports, or even riding a horse - and the bleeding almost always stops on its own. If you're thinking of having sex with your boyfriend in the future, you should make sure you understand how your body works first. That way, you can make informed choices and protect yourself from STIs and pregnancy.

Pregnancy Prevention

I was thinking about going on the Pill, but I want to know how it works first. Are there any side effects? Is it harmful?

It's great that you're taking this decision so seriously. You want to feel comfortable about your birth control method and being informed is essential. The Pill mainly works by preventing the release of eggs from the ovaries. But in some cases, an egg is still released. That's when the Pill's other effects are called into action: The Pill also keeps the lining of the uterus thin, which helps to prevent a fertilized egg from growing inside the uterus. It also helps keep sperm from reaching an egg by changing the cervical mucus and slowing the movements of the fallopian tubes.

Common side effects include some nausea during the first month, mild spotting between periods, and a little weight gain. More serious side effects, which are rare and occur mostly in women over age 35 and in smokers – include blood clots in your legs, heart attacks, and stroke. Gallbladder problems and non-cancerous liver tumors are also a risk.

But there are benefits to the Pill too. Periods are more regular and less painful and there is a lower chance of ectopic pregnancies (pregnancies that grow outside the uterus in the fallopian tubes) and pelvic inflammatory disease (when an STI becomes severe). The Pill may also help prevent ovarian and uterine cancers. The best plan is to discuss the pros and cons with your doctor.

Lately, my boyfriend and I have gotten pretty serious. We both want to wait until we're married to have sex, so we were thinking of going through the motions of sex, but leaving our clothes on. Can sperm get through?

Here's the deal: Sex is sex – with clothes off or on. So having sex with your clothes on not only counts as intercourse, but it also puts you at risk for getting pregnant or catching sexually transmitted infections. Fabrics have millions of tiny holes where sperm, bacteria, or viruses can sneak through – just hold your shirt or your underwear up to a bright light and see for yourself. That's why condoms are made of latex or other materials which don't allow stuff to pass through. So if you and your boyfriend have sex with your clothes on, there's a chance you'll get pregnant – not something you'll want to risk. A safer bet would be to abstain from sex completely or practice safe sex by using a condom.

I'm 15 and I want to go on the pill, but I can't ask my parents because they¹ll think I'm going around having sex with everyone. How can I get on birth control without my parent's consent? I don't want to make an appointment, either, because I'm scared they'll call my house. Help!

In most states, there underage teens are legally allowed to get birth control and pregnancy testing without their parents' knowledge or permission. These confidentiality laws were created to support teens being responsible for their sexual activity even if their parents aren't supportive. But not all doctors are aware of them or feel comfortable keeping information from a parent who is demanding this kind of information.

Obviously, it would be easiest if you could talk to your parents about these kinds of things, but most teenagers aren't lucky enough to have those kinds of parents. If you feel comfortable talking to your pediatrician or family doctor about birth control and they agree to respect your privacy, that might be the easiest thing to do. Your health insurance company will likely mail bills to your parents with the names of doctors you see and any tests that were ordered, so be prepared to answer questions about why you went to the doctor.

If you're absolutely paranoid about your parents finding out, your best bet would be to find out if the local county health department has a teen or call Planned Parenthood. Many larger hospitals have adolescent clinics that are also used to dealing with your kind of situation. Find out how much an appointment costs and if they have a "sliding scale" for people who can't pay the full price. They will need a phone number and address to reach you in case of abnormal tests results. You may want to consider asking a relative, older sibling, or friend to let you use their contact information for privacy.

I had sex about a month ago. We used a condom and I did get my period, but it was lighter than usual. Can a girl get her period even if she's pregnant?

It is not unusual to have bleeding that can look like a period during pregnancy. Condoms are only about 88% effective in preventing pregnancy based on how people actually use them (not perfect use), but they are still the best protection again STIs. So you can't rule out pregnancy as a possible cause for your light period. You can do a home pregnancy test but you might want to check with your doctor instead – she'll do a pregnancy test and, if it is negative, she'll be able to give you helpful birth control advice.

If you do find out you're pregnant and you don't know who to turn to, find your local Planned Parenthood for confidential info and support. Call 1-800-230-PLAN or go online to plannedparenthood.org.

I'm thinking of having sex with my boyfriend and I'm wondering what time of the month is most safe in terms of <u>not</u> getting pregnant?

There is not time that is absolutely, guaranteed, 100 percent safe. The truth is you can only get pregnant when an egg leaves your ovaries (which is called ovulation) and that happens somewhere in the middle of your cycle. The problem is no one knows for sure when this 48 hour ovulation period begins and when it ends. Even if your periods are very regular, the number of days between each one probably isn't exactly the same each month. Neither is the time you ovulate. If you have sex a few days before you ovulate, sperm can live inside the uterus for five days and can be there when an egg finally comes along. And that means you can get pregnant!

Guessing about your cycle is way too risky a form of birth control. A better way to prevent pregnancy is to always use a condom with spermicidal foam or jelly, which will help kill any sperm that might escape.

My best friend just told me that when she and her boyfriend were having sex, the condom broke. The next day, she went to a clinic and took the morning after pill. I'm not really sure what that is.

Don't feel bad about not knowing about the "morning after pill" – known more accurately as Emergency Contraception (ECP) because it is effective up to 72 hours (3 days) after an episode of unprotected sex. It is one of the best kept secrets in medicine. This strategy has been used in emergency rooms for decades for rape victims, to help cut down the chance of becoming pregnant. Doctors used to prescribe large doses of some birth control pills as ECP, but now there are two prescription medications made just for this purpose. It is NOT an abortion pill and will not cause an abortion if it is taken by someone who is already pregnant.

Think of ECP as what to do if your condom breaks so that you don't get pregnant. If condoms are all that you are using for birth control, know that accidents do happen and ECP can cut the chance of getting pregnant by about 85% from a single episode of unprotected sex. It works by preventing ovulation and by changing the lining of the uterus so a fertilized egg won't stick to it. The pills can make you nauseated so many women take motion-sickness medication with it.

So, if your condom breaks (or if you made a mistake and didn't use one) and you don't want to get pregnant, call your doctor and ask for ECP. If you don't have a doctor, you can call the national Emergency Contraception Hotline to find a doctor who will prescribe it for you – 1-888-NOT-2-LATE. Just remember, the sooner you take it, the better it works. And if you're finding that your condoms break often, you should think about using something in addition to condoms, like a hormonal form of birth control (pills, injection, or vaginal ring).

Can you get pregnant if you have sex while you're having your period?

Believe it or not, you *can* get pregnant during your period. In fact, there is *no* safe time to have unprotected sex. It's true that women are less likely to ovulate (release an egg) while menstruating, but it is possible. And you don't have to ovulating at the exact time you're having sex in order to get pregnant. An egg is good for up to 48 hours after it's released and sperm can live up to five days in a vagina, uterus and fallopian tubes. So it is possible to get pregnant several days after having sex. The bottom line is that you should always use a condom, even during your period. During that time of the month, the risk of catching HIV and Hepatitis B are higher than usual with unprotected sex because of the direct exposure to blood. One more thing to keep in mind – condoms have a greater chance of slipping off if you have sex during your period, so you might want to wait to have sex until your period is over.

My friend thinks she's pregnant. Besides not getting your period, what are some other signs of pregnancy?

Pregnancies vary from person to person – and a woman may have all, some, or none of the signs other women experience. Here are the most common early signs of pregnancy: breast tenderness/fullness, nausea, feeling very tired and sleeping more often, and frequent urination. Lower abdominal pains and weight gain can also occur as the pregnancy progresses, but not usually until about a month after a period is missed.

If your friend's period is one or more weeks late, tell her to take a home pregnancy test because it should be positive by then. If the test is negative and she still hasn't gotten her period a week later, she should see a doctor. The earlier a pregnancy is detected, the more time she'll have to consider her options.

I'm thinking about going on the Pill, but I've heard it can have side effects, like weight gain and acne. Is this true?

Everybody responds differently to the Pill – and many don't notice any side effects. It's true that the hormones in birth control pills can affect other parts of your body. Some girls and women retain water or feel hungrier on when they are taking the Pill. Exercising and cutting back on salt will make you feel less bloated and watching what you snack on can help keep your weight in check. While the hormones in some birth control pills can make sebaceous glands go haywire - causing breakouts, doctors often prescribe newer forms of birth control pills to *clear up* acne. Other common side effects include nausea, headaches, and bleeding between your cycles, but these usually go away within a few months of starting the Pill. If the side effects don't get better or you notice symptoms that you're concerned about, tell your doctor. There are many kinds of birth control pills so you might have to try a different version of the Pill to find the one that's best for you

I always thought that the Pill was an effective form of birth control, but my friend recently told me I can still get pregnant even if I'm taking the Pill. Is she right?

No form of birth control, other than not having sex, is 100% guaranteed to prevent pregnancy. But the Pill comes pretty close - it's over 99% effective if used properly. That last part's the kicker: "if used properly." The Pill becomes less effective if you forget to take it at the same time each day, miss doses and have to double up, get sick and throw up right after taking it, or are also taking certain other mediations or herbal supplements. (Check with your doctor or pharmacist to find out if you're taking anything that could interfere.) But here's something major to keep in mind: while the Pill can be a super way to prevent getting pregnant, it does not protect you against STIs. So, if you pair the Pill with a condom, not only will you increase your chances of not getting pregnant, you'll also protect yourself against HIV and other infections.

My boyfriend says I can't get pregnant if we keep our underwear on when we fool around. Is he right?

You definitely could get pregnant any time your boyfriend's sperm gets near the opening of your vagina – even if you're not having intercourse. Sperm are strong swimmers and they're on a mission to find your eggs. Wearing underwear while having sex doesn't do anything to prevent pregnancy. Underwear is nothing more than a weave of fibers, which leaves plenty of room for sperm and STI-causing bacteria to slip through. (Don't believe it? Put a drop of water on a pair of panties and watch how fast it leaks through.) To be safe, keep your clothes on and don't have sex. But if you're having sex or being intimate with your boyfriend, always use a condom to prevent pregnancy and STIs.

Is there any kind of birth control that is 100 percent effective? I'm really freaked out about getting pregnant!

The only type of birth control that is 100 percent effective is *not having sex*. Birth control pills and shots are pretty effective at preventing pregnancy (although they don't protect against STIs). But even if you take them exactly as you're supposed to, there's still about a one percent chance of getting pregnant.

You can decrease your risk by using condoms along with birth control pills or other forms of hormonal contraception. But don't pair up a male and female condom, because the friction can cause tears and decrease the effectiveness. And don't double up on male condoms either – they can slide off or rip, leaving you with much less protection than as single condom.

If you're not ready to cope with the consequences of having sex you might want to consider holding off for a while – it's a lot easier than dealing with an unplanned pregnancy. There's no such thing as totally safe sex, so make sure you're ready to deal with the risk before you do it.

My boyfriend and I were going to have sex, but after only a few seconds we decided not to and he pulled out. But now my period is a few days late. I couldn't be pregnant from only a few seconds, right?

I'm afraid you're actually wrong about that. There is no amount of unprotected sex that is guaranteed not to get you pregnant – so even if you only had sex for a split second, you *are* at risk for pregnancy and STIs. This is why it's important to get out a condom *before* you start messing around.

If your periods are usually regular, you may want to take a pregnancy test. Some other early signs of pregnancy include feeling tired all the time, breast tenderness and nausea (especially in the mornings). A positive home pregnancy test after a late period is pretty accurate, but if the test is negative it should be repeated a few days later. And you should see a doctor for an official test if your period is two weeks late, even if a home pregnancy test is negative.

I have a serious boyfriend and I'm thinking of going on the Pill. How long does it take to become effective? Also, how important is it to take it at the same time every day?

Birth control pills help prevent pregnancy by releasing hormones that keep ovaries from ovulating (releasing eggs). But it can take up to a month after you start taking the Pill for those hormones to do their job effectively, so you should use condoms with the Pill for at least that long. Because the Pill prevents pregnancy but not HIV or other STIs, you should continue using a condom to prevent infections while using birth control pills for better pregnancy prevention.

Another reason to be careful that first month on the Pill: it's important to take your birth control pills at the same time every day and it can take a while to get used to doing that. Oral contraceptives control your home levels day-by-day. If you take a pill in the morning one day then wait until the next night to take the next done, you'll increase your chance of ovulating – and possibly becoming pregnant. Try keeping your birth control pills near your toothbrush so you think about taking them when you brush your teeth at bedtime. Or set a daily alarm on your phone to remind you to take your pills at a certain time.

Don't freak if you forget to take a pill, though. Just take it as soon as you remember, then take the next pill at your usually time (even if it means taking two pills at once) and be extra careful with your condoms for the rest of the month. If you miss more than one pill, don't take more than two at a time to catch up – the hormones in more than a double dose may make upset your stomach and make you vomit. If you miss two days, take two pills one day and two pills the next day. Then you'll be back on track with one pill a day by the third day. If you miss your pill for three days, you are going to get your period because you missed too many pills - so stop taking the current pack of pills, wait for you period and start the next pack on the first day of your next period.

My friend had unprotected sex and she thinks she's pregnant. How long should she wait before she takes an at-home test? If she is pregnant, will it show up the next day?

No, it will not show up that soon. Urine pregnancy test should be accurate anywhere from 10 to 14 days after someone gets pregnant, but not before then. So after two weeks, she can take a test – just make sure she follows the directions carefully. And remember, it's never 100 percent accurate.

If the test is positive – even if the line or mark is faint – she should see a doctor right away. If it is negative she should repeat the test a week later if she still hasn't had her period. Better yet, she should see a doctor, explain that she had unprotected sex, and get a thorough checkup. The doctor will do a urine pregnancy test or order a blood pregnancy test, which can detect pregnancies earlier.

In most states, anyone 17 or older can buy emergency contraception pills from the pharmacy without a prescription – but it needs to be taken within 72 hours (3 days) after unprotected sex to reduce the chance of pregnancy. If you are younger than 17 years old, you will need to see a doctor to get a prescription. Anyone can call the emergency contraception hotline for more information and locations where emergency contraception is sold: 1-888-NOT-2-LATE.

My boyfriend told me it's almost impossible to get pregnant the first time you have sex, because your hymen hasn't broken yet so it's hard for the sperm to get through. Is that true?

The hymen isn't a security guard at the entrance of the vagina! In most women, it is only a slightly thickened ring of tissue – kind of like how a balloon has a rolled up edge on the part you blow into, which makes the opening slightly smaller. Lots of women believe the myth that you can't get pregnant the first time you have sex and, unfortunately, several of them have found out the hard way that it isn't true. You need to use protection each and every time you have sex to protect yourself from pregnancy and STIs!

Hymens come in all shapes and sizes and many women who have never had sex can rip or stretch their hymens during exercise. Some women never tear their hymen during intercourse – their hymens are stretchy enough that they don't rip. Other women have hymens that are so tight they can't have sex, but this can be taken care of by a doctor.

I took a home pregnancy test and it came out negative. But the directions say not to take the test until after the first day of your missed period. Mine's not due for another week. Could I be pregnant?

Because you're not due for your period yet, it's possible for you to be pregnant but it is too early to detect it with urine tests. But don't freak out until you take the test again – once you know you've missed your period. This is why doctors will always ask you when the first day of your last period was – it's the best way to guess if someone may be pregnant.

Why do you need to wait? It takes about two weeks after you become pregnant for the level or pregnancy hormone in your urine to be high enough to show up on the test. And on average, you period starts about two weeks after ovulation, which is the time you're most likely to get pregnant. Even if you follow the directions and the test still comes out negative, wait a week and repeat it if your period still hasn't arrived.

What kind of birth control are you using? Using a birth control method correctly helps cut back on the fear that you may not get your period each month. Everyone can buy condoms, but if you aren't sure how to use them or if you also want a kind of birth control that is better at preventing pregnancy, see a doctor.

My boyfriend and I are thinking of having sex, and we plan to use a condom. But I want to talk to my mom about helping me get birth control pills so we can be extra-safe. I know my mom wouldn't be angry with me, but my boyfriend doesn't want me to ask her because he's worried that she'll make me stop seeing him. Should I listen to him?

It's always best to talk about important issues like sex and birth control with a parent or guardian if you can. Unfortunately, most teenagers know the subject will upset their parents or aren't sure how they'd react. If you think you're lucky enough to have the kind of mom who will be supportive, you should tell her.

Adding a hormonal form of birth control to condoms definitely improves pregnancy prevention compared with condoms alone. Condoms are the best option for preventing sexually transmitted infections, but for pregnancy prevention they are only about 88% effective if used correctly each time. You can also increase pregnancy prevention by adding spermicidal foam, jelly, or inserts with condoms, but it isn't as effective as using a hormonal method of birth control with condoms. Luckily, there are so many choices of birth control for young women these days – injections (monthly or every 3 months), pills, patches, vaginal rings. The trick is to find one that best works with your body and to use it exactly as directed.

My boyfriend and I don't want to have sex, but we want to closer physically. A friend suggested we should try "dry sex." What exactly is this? Can you get pregnant from it if you're both fully clothed? What if you just have underwear on? Please help - I don't know who else I can talk to about this.

"Dry sex" usually means rubbing against each other, fully clothed, as if you were having sex. Your chances are seriously slim of getting pregnant this way, but it's not totally impossible, since semen can pass through clothing. So, the less clothing you're wearing, the riskier it is. Keep in mind that getting so intimate with your boyfriend may lead to other things, so make sure you both know your limits *before* you find yourself in the middle of a make out session.

My boyfriend and I had sex without a condom, but he pulled out before he was done. He promised me that it's totally safe that way, but I'm worried. Could I still get pregnant?

You boyfriend shouldn't make promises he can't keep! "Pulling out" is another term of the withdrawal method of birth control and it doesn't work for a couple of reasons. Before a guy ejaculates, there is a small amount of seminal fluid that leaks from his penis. The fluid *does* contain sperm, so if you're unprotected, you're definitely putting yourself at risk - it only takes one strong sperm swimmer for a pregnancy to happen.

It's also way too easy for a guy to misjudge his timing and pull out too late. The best way to avoid pregnancy is to always use condoms, along with contraceptive jelly, the Pill or another method of hormonal birth control (injections or vaginal ring).

STI Safe or Scary?

I heard that you can catch genital warts from sitting on public toilet seats. Is that true? Yuck!

Genital warts are indeed yucky but it's really hard to catch *anything* from a public toilet seat unless you were really trying. Think about it – the part of your body that touches the toilet seat is the edges of your butt and your upper thighs. You'd have to do some strange wiggling around in order to get direct contact with your genital area!

Sexually transmitted infections are spread by viruses and bacteria, most of which don't survive for very long outside a human body. Toilet seats with urine, blood or other body fluids allow viruses and bacteria to last a little longer, until the temperature gets too cold or they dry up. You should always take advantage of the toilet seat covers in public bathroom – they provide enough protection again everything except a soaking wet toilet seat. If there is no toilet seat cover, toilet paper is just as good. And if the toilet seat is wet but you really need to pee, you can always squat over the seat without actually sitting down to keep your bottom from touching it. Just make sure that you don't miss the bowl – you don't want to leave a wet seat for the next person!

If you kiss someone who has AIDS and you have a cut in your mouth, can you get it?

There have been no known cases of HIV transmission through exposure to saliva only. But technically it *is* possible to contract HIV through kissing. Scientists still don't know people's exact chance of getting HIV that way but we do know that HIV is spread through contact with body fluids and the greater the exposure to these fluids, the higher the risk of spreading the virus. Also, body fluids like blood, semen, and vaginal discharge can have more virus particles in them than saliva and sweat. So having unprotected sex is much more risky than French kissing. And French kissing with a cut in your mouth is riskier than if you weren't cut because there's exposure to your blood. Closed, "dry mouth" kissing is considered safe. If you have kissed someone with HIV and are concerned about it, you should consider getting tested.

My boyfriend and I have talked about having oral sex. Can you get pregnant or an STI from that? Is it safer if you don't swallow the sperm?

First of all, you can't get pregnant from oral sex – there's no way for the sperm to reach your eggs that way. But you *can* catch a whole bunch of STIs from unprotected oral sex, whether the semen is swallowed or not. Infections like HIV, hepatitis B, hepatitis C and syphilis are all spread through body fluids and blood. And since everyone has tiny cuts in their gums and tongues from brushing their teeth and chewing food (even if you don't feel them or notice any bleeding), these infections can travel from semen into your body. Other STIs, like gonorrhea, herpes, Chlamydia, and even human papillomavirus (which causes genital warts) are not spread through the bloodstream but they could possibly cause infections in your mouth and throat from unprotected sex.

So if you do have oral sex, use a condom on your boyfriend and a dental dam (a thin square piece of latex) on yourself to prevent STIs during oral sex. And if you can't find a dental dam at a pharmacy you can make one by getting a condom, snipping off the tip, cutting it lengthwise, and opening it into a rectangle, which then goes over your private parts.

I've been seeing this guy for a few months, but I've barely seen him this summer. The other day, I went to the beach and kissed another guy. I know if you have sex with someone else, you should always tell your boyfriend because of STIs and stuff, but does the same rule apply to kissing? I mean, there's no way I could get an STI from kissing, right?

It's true that you can catch some STIs from kissing, but it's definitely less risky than having sex with someone. You can catch skin-to-skin infections spread by viruses, like herpes and warts, by kissing your grandmother or sharing lip balm just as easily as by kissing a guy. Infections like gonorrhea and Chlamydia live deeper in people's throats, so you're not likely to catch them if you don't do some serious making out.

So, should you tell your boyfriend? If you feel guilty about doing it, it's probably a good idea to tell him, but I don't think that any doctor would recommend it for medical reasons. Unlike testing genitals for STIs, tests for the same infections in different areas aren't recommended before starting a relationship with someone new.

My boyfriend and I have been fooling around a lot lately, and even though we haven't had sex, I'm worried about catching an STI. I know he hasn't had sex with anyone else, so that means I'm totally safe, right?

First of all, you can never really know if your partner has never had sex with anyone else unless you've followed them around every minute of their whole life. Many people deny that they've been sexually active in the past because they think it would make them less appealing to you. This can happen with older partners who think you may be worried about being less experienced sexually than he is or that you won't be concerned about catching an STI from him if he's a virgin. It could also happen if your partner was sexually molested as a child – it's something they tend to block out and deny ever happened. So unless you've seen him with another partner, how would you actually know the truth? This is why you need to protect yourself from STIs with every partner, regardless of what they tell you.

You do not have to have intercourse with someone to catch an STI from him or her. Infections like herpes and genital warts are spread by skin-to-skin contact only – no sex is required. It is possible to spread infections like gonorrhea and Chlamydia without going all the way and many STIs spread by genital sex can also be spread by oral sex.

My friend says you can catch an STI from swimming in a pool with a guy who has an infection. Is that true?

Pools are rarely the source of an infection for several reasons. There is so much water in a pool compared to the amount of infectious material from someone with an STI or any kind of infected wound that it would be diluted very much. It's kind of like what would happen if you emptied one packet of Kool-Aid into a pool – it would be so scattered in the water that it wouldn't change the color or flavor at all. Most types of bacteria and viruses also won't grow if there is enough chlorine in the pool or if the water temperature is below normal body temperature. It may be easier to spread sexually transmitted infections in hot tubs because there is less water, the water temperature is better for growing bacteria, and people tend to not use enough chlorine in them.

If you use a condom, does that mean you're totally protected from STIs?

Condoms are definitely the best protection against STIs available, but they won't protect you 100%. They work by preventing skin-to-skin contact but there's quite a bit of skin that a condom doesn't cover. That's why condoms can still allow infections like herpes, genital warts, and syphilis to spread from person to person. And, condoms can rip or slip off, leaving you completely unprotected from both STIs and pregnancy.

If you've decided to have sex, talk with your partner first. Ask about previous partners and if they've ever had an infection before - but realize that you may not get the truth if your partner is worried that the answer may scare you off. Some couples schedule appointments for STI testing together before having sex the first time. This is a good idea, but testing isn't usually done for herpes and genital warts if none are seen during the visit.

I hooked up with this guy a few weeks ago and now I have these itchy bumps around my vagina. We didn't go all the way, so I can't have an STI, right?

First, the good news: it's possible that those bumps came from something as minor as razor burn (if you shave down there), irritation from tight underwear, or an allergic reaction to your laundry detergent. The bad news is that you *could* have a sexually transmitted infection (STI), so you need to see a doctor right away. Two common STIs you can catch without going all the way are human papilloma virus (HPV) which causes genital warts, and herpes simplex virus (HSV). They spread through skin-to-skin contact – especially between moist regions like the mouth and genital areas. There are some other STIs that spread through body fluids, which means that oral sex and even French kissing can be risky. To help protect yourself against infection, always, always use a condom, even if you're fooling around without going all the way. It won't guarantee you won't catch something, but it can help reduce the risk.

What is herpes and how can I avoid it?

Herpes simplex is a virus that can affect your lips (as "cold sores" or your genitals as a sexually transmitted infection). Flare ups, which happen most often when you're stressed or sick, start off as a group of blisters which burst and leave a red open sore,. Herpes is very contagious – sores on the lips can spread genital herpes to another person and vice versa. There's no cure, but medications can make the outbreaks shorter.

Herpes blisters heal very well, so you can't tell if a guy has ever had it just by looking at his skin. That's why it's important to be comfortable talking to your boyfriend about STIs before having sex. The best way to avoid genital herpes is to avoid skin-to-skin contact during sex. Condoms help, but they don't cover enough area to give you total protection. If your boyfriend has the herpes virus, *never* have sex during an outbreak. And don't assume you're safe just because you don't see sores on his skin – herpes is the most contagious about a day *before* the blisters appear.

My boyfriend and I have fooled around but haven't had sex. He's a virgin, so that means I'm totally safe from STIs, right?

Not necessarily. Infections like herpes and genital warts are spread by skin-to-skin contact only – no sex required. And oral sex (where a person stimulates their partner's genitals with their mouth) can spread almost as many STIs as sexual intercourse. Also, keep in mind that some guys will lie about their sexual history to make you feel more comfortable, so it's impossible to

134

be 100% sure what he has or hasn't done. That's why, when things get hot and heavy, it's vital to use a condom to protect yourself from STIs, no matter how safe you think you are.

I noticed bumps near my vagina. My boyfriend and I have been having sex for a year, but he says I was his first so I can't have an STI, right?

The good news: lots of things can cause those bumps, from ingrown hairs to having sex without enough lubrication. The bad news: only your doctor can tell for sure whether you're STI-free.

When it comes to infections like herpes and genital warts, skin-to-skin contact is all it takes. So even if your boyfriend was a virgin when he met you, he could have pick up one of these viral infections from a past makeout session. While it's best to discuss your sexual history with your boyfriend before you do the deed, you can't count on the info to protect you from STIs.

Unfortunately, there's a slim chance that your boyfriend isn't being completely straight with you about his sexual past. He could be afraid that you'd think less of him if you find out he's had sex before or has cheated on you. And if he suspects he has an STI, he may be too embarrassed to tell you.

Obviously, you should use a condom no matter what. The best way to find out what's up with the bumps is to see your doctor.

I'm sexually active and I've started to notice small bumps along my vaginal area. It also burns when I pee. Is there any place I can get checked without my parents knowing?

It's good that you want to get tested right away to find out what's causing these problems. While your symptoms could be from something other than a sexually transmitted infection (STI), you can't tell for sure. And since you're having sex, you need to get checked out to be totally sure. In fact, even if you had no symptoms at all, it's recommended that sexually active teens be tested for STIs at least once a year.

Most states in the US have laws that allow minors to be checked and treated for STIs without their parents' permission or knowledge. These laws exist because politicians realized that many teens can't tell their parents that they are having sex. And if teens couldn't seek treatment on their own, STIs would become an even bigger problem than they already are. To find a place near you, search online for your local department of health clinics or see if there's a Planned Parenthood in your area. You can also call the Center for Disease Control's National STD Hotline at 800-227-8922 or use the clinic locator online at GetTested.cdc.gov

Sexual Situations

I made out with my boyfriend the other night, and now my inner thighs are sore. We didn't have sex, but I'm worried. Should I see a doctor?

Ever do a lot of exercise without stretching out first? Ouch, right? Unless you're used to twisting yourself into a pretzel regularly, all that rolling around and wrapping legs around each other can lead to some serious muscle cramps. It sounds like you pulled a muscle, so treat it like any other muscle strain. Soak in a warm bath or use a heating pad to warm up the muscles. Then, if you can stand it, take it easy on your thighs (and your guy) for a few days.

I just started dating this guy and I'm worried that he's going to expect me to have sex pretty soon. The thing is I'm still a virgin and I'm really scared to do it. I'm not even sure I want to. How can I say no and not lose him as my boyfriend?

Kudos to you for being smart enough to know that sex is nothing to take lightly – especially if it's your first time. There are tons of emotions involved, so unless you feel totally comfortable with your boyfriend – and with your own decision – you could end up feeling hurt or vulnerable afterwards. That's why it's crucial to be really open with your boyfriend about how physical you want to get with him. If you sense that your relationship is getting more physical, or that he's got sex on his mind, don't wait until you're in the middle of making out to bring it up to him. Next time you're chatting about your relationship, tell him that you want to take the physical side of things slow because it's a really big deal to you and you need to be completely ready. Then be clear about what stuff you are – and aren't- cool about doing. Most likely, he'll respect you for it – and more importantly, you'll respect yourself for being honest with him. (And, by the way, if your boyfriend gets angry or pressures you, he's so not worthy of you.)

Last week, during a really heavy makeout session, my boyfriend was touching me a lot down there, and I ended up bleeding a little. Is this anything to worry about?

Don't worry. It sounds like your boyfriend may have been touching your hymen, the thin rim of skin around the opening to the vagina. When this area gets stretched by fingers, penises, or strenuous exercise there can be a little bleeding. The bleeding can make you a little nervous but it's not dangerous and stops on its own.

My boyfriend and I started having sex a few months ago, but I've never had an orgasm. Am I doing something wrong?

First, a definition: an orgasm is the climax of sexual excitement. In men, ejaculation often happens with an orgasm – but not always.

Unlike men, many women have to learn to develop their orgasmic response. This often requires that you find out what is pleasurable for you and how you like to be touched. It's also important to feel comfortable with your partner and want to have sex. Fear of getting pregnant or being caught having sex can prevent you from relaxing enough from having an orgasm. Focusing on orgasms as such an important thing also can distract you from fully enjoying a sexual experience.

Sometimes I feel like I have to pee when my boyfriend and I fool around. Is that normal?

What you are describing sounds like irritation of the urethra, the opening to the bladder. (The urethra can be easy to miss if you're looking in a mirror – it's a small hole north of the vaginal opening.) The friction from sex can cause this problem, but it usually goes away soon afterwards. If you are allergic to the spermicide on condoms, you can have some irritation that comes and goes after sex. Some STIs can also cause this symptom, but it's more likely to bother you at other times too.

Because it's only a short distance from the urethra to the bladder, women can get urine infections from skin bacteria making the trip up there. This is why all women should pee after sex (and, if you can, before too). Bladder infections can cause painful urination, a feeling that your bladder isn't completely empty after peeing, or the need to pee more often and urgently. While the symptoms could be mild at first, if left untreated they can lead to a more serious infection of the kidneys. It's probably a good idea for you to get checked out by a doctor to make sure everything is ok.

I've had sex three times and the last time, I bled. I thought that only happened your first time. Is there something wrong with me?

There is probably nothing wrong with you. I know it seems weird, but it's not unusual for girls to bleed the first few times they have sex. Some girls don't bleed at all, some bleed once, and some bleed a bunch of times. So most likely, there's nothing to worry about. The bleeding could be caused by friction during intercourse, so you might want to use a lubricated condom or extra lubrication added to cut down on any irritation. If you experience severe bleeding or if it continues to happen each time you have sex, it could be something else, like a sexually transmitted infection. To put your mind at east, it's a good idea to see your doctor or go to a Planned Parenthood office just to make sure everything is okay. You can find the nearest Planned Parenthood office online at plannedparenthood.org or their hotline – 800-230-PLAN.

I'm a virgin and my boyfriend is not. When we tried to have sex recently, it hurt me so much that I told him to stop. What's wrong with me?

Relax. The first time is usually a little scary and uncomfortable. If your vaginal opening is still surrounded by a thin piece of skin called the hymen, a penis can stretch or rip it. For some girls, this hurts, a few bleed a little and some feel no pain at all. Usually, if you're really excited, your vagina relaxes and lubricates itself to make intercourse easier. Stressing about it a lot may keep this from happening – and could be your "I'm not ready" alarm telling you to slow down. Think about whether you're making the right move and tell your boyfriend that this is a big step for you. If you do have sex, suing a lubricated latex condom and a water-based lubricant may help. Don't use anything oil-based for lubrication (like petroleum jelly or lotion) because it can damage a condom. Whether or not the pain continues, you should see a doctor for a gynecological exam once you start having sex.

Lately, I've been masturbating before I go to bed. It feels really good, but I've heard that doing it too often can be dangerous. Is that right? Can my doctor tell whether or not I'm touching myself?

First, let's get one thing totally straight. Masturbation is a completely normal way of exploring your own body. Most people do it – even babies and children touch themselves – although most people feel weird talking about it. For some reason, many folks are taught from an early age that masturbation is something they should avoid and be ashamed of. That is probably due to all the crazy myths out there. Masturbation will not cause zits, make you go crazy, or give you hairy palms.

In fact, there is nothing dangerous or dirty about masturbation. It's the safest sex anyone can have, since there's no risk of getting pregnant or catching a sexually transmitted infection. It's a much healthier way of dealing with stress than using drugs or heavy alcohol drinking and it helps many people relax before sleep. And don't worry – NOBODY (not your friends or even your doctor) has any way of knowing whether or not you masturbate.

What exactly is a G-spot?

G-spot was named after Dr. Grafenberg, the doctor who first described it. It is a bump of tissue inside the vagina, the size of a quarter or less that is more sensitive than the surrounding area. It is usually on the front wall of the vagina and about two inches inside.

Stimulating the G-spot can help lead to orgasms, which is why people talk about the importance of "finding the G-spot." But it is only one of several extra-sensitive spots on a woman's body. It's good to be aware of where such sensitive spots are, but for some women they aren't that much more sensitive. Just as not everyone likes the same color or flavor of ice cream, stimulating the G-spot in some people isn't as good as focusing on other spots that you and your partner discover yourselves.

Many women find that once they are able to bring themselves to orgasm, they are able to achieve orgasms with their partners. There are several books on this subject that may give you some useful suggestions.

Is it ever not okay to touch yourself?

Your body is yours, so technically you're free to explore your own body whenever you want. Masturbation does not cause acne or hairy palms, but could become a problem if you do it all the time instead of other things (like studying or spending time with friends).

There are some basic rules for masturbation. Touching yourself in public makes other people feel uncomfortable and could get you arrested because it is illegal. Limit it to times and places when you're alone or with someone you're comfortable with. Only touch yourself with hands or objects that are clean. Skin in the genital area is thin, so friction from rubbing can lead to small scrapes and infections. Also make sure you don't have jagged nails or touch yourself with something rough. Some STIs can be spread with sex toys, so never share them with others.

My boyfriend and I have agreed we're not ready for sex yet, but now he's asking me to have oral sex with him instead. I don't feel comfortable with the idea, but I'm afraid if I tell him I'm not ready, he might get tired of me and start going out with someone more experienced. He says he loves me, but if I say no, he might change his mind. Please help!

Ask yourself why you're not ready yet. You might be embarrassed by the idea of oral sex (which is when you use your mouth to stimulate the other person's genitals) or worried that you'll do something wrong. Or maybe you're just not ready to get that close to someone. If you tell him *why* you're not into it, he'll realize it's not because you don't care about him.

You may be nervous about telling your guy how you feel, but if he really loves you, he'll totally respect your decision. And if he's not supportive, why would you want to be with him anyway? Any guy who ditches you just because you won't fool around with him is pretty sleazy. You deserve a guy who will wait until you feel comfortable – and there are plenty of guys like that out there.

I had sex with my boyfriend a few times but I don't want to do it anymore. I don't know how to tell him without hurting his feelings. What should I do?

Just because you had sex doesn't mean you have to keep doing it – you can change your mind at any time. As long as you give your guy concrete reasons for your decision he'll realize it has nothing to do with how you feel about him. Try saying something like "I thought I was ready to handle the risks, but now I feel it's just too much stress for me at the moment." After all, only *you* can decide if you're ready for sex. If he cares about you, he will respect any decision you make.

My friends talk about getting to first and second base. What do they mean?

The old baseball analogy is still around... No one knows who decided to assign a base for every sexual conquest, but it's been around for a long time and it was probably a guy. There are also some variations if you ask different people.

Everyone agrees that the first base is kissing – some say only the French kind. At second base, a girl's breasts are touched – either over or under her shirt. When a couple makes it to third, touching of the private parts has occurred. Although oral sex isn't actually on the baseball diamond, it is probably somewhere between third base and home base. And a home run is going all the way by having intercourse. Although the game talk may be silly, a lot of people think it's a good way of discussing sex without being embarrassed by using technical words.

I've heard my friends talking about orgasms, but I have no idea what they are - and I'm way too embarrassed to ask. How do I know whether or not I've had one?

Okay, here's the deal in a nutshell: When you're fooling around with someone (or touching yourself), it's possible to get so turned on that your body sort of takes over. Blood rushes to your genitals, your skin becomes super sensitive and the muscles all over your body begin to tense up. If the tension builds to a certain level, your body may release it in a wave of contractions in your uterus and vagina and – ta-da! – you have an orgasm. (This is what people mean when they talk about "coming.") The experience is different for everyone and it's usually associated with ejaculation in guys.

It's tough to say what an orgasm feels like, so you may have had one without knowing it. Most women describe a warm, tingling feeling in their private parts, then twitching contractions followed by a pleasant, relaxed feeling. Don't stress about whether or not you've had one. Women's magazines may hype them up to sound like everyone's having them, but it will happen when you're comfortable and the time is right.

This is really embarrassing, but I don't know who else I can ask about this. I was looking around on the internet, and I accidentally clicked on a porn site! I closed the screen right away, but it kind of turned me on. I've actually thought about looking for it again.

There is a reason that there is so much pornography on cable, on the web and in magazines – sexual images are sexually stimulating and all of us humans are sexual creatures. These days almost everyone has wound up on a porn site by making a typo in a web address. But there are some important things to consider when looking at porn online. First, laws are different in each state, but in most places you have to be over 18 to have access to pornographic images. Clicking on the "I'm over 18" when you're not can cause you legal trouble. Second, child pornography is always illegal and downloading or sending such images can get you arrested. Third, a computer may keep cookies or links to these sites on the computer and your boss, friends and family could see what you've been looking at. This could get you into a whole different kind of trouble with work and personal relationships. And downloading these images to the computer, by accident or on purpose, makes it even easier.

I had a dream I had sex with a girl. Could I be gay?

It's absolutely normal to have romantic dreams about people of the same sex even if you're not gay. Besides, if you are gay it's unlikely that you'd only feel attracted to other girls while you sleep. Sex in dreams may represent actual sex or just be a way of showing affection for someone you care about.

Dreams are the way your mind deals with all the information it has received while you were awake. This is why you often dream about people you have strong emotional feelings towards or about something you saw on television during the day. It's also common for a character in a dream to start off as one person and turn into a different person later on, or for one person to represent another in your dream. But no matter what they mean, dreams can't determine your sexual preference.

I went to a party the other night and passed out after a few drinks. When I woke up, I felt awful – but even scarier, I was really sore down there. I'm afraid I might have been given a date-rape drug! Is there any way I can tell?

If you think you might have been slipped a date-rape drug, see your doctor right away. The longer you wait, the less likely a blood test can tell if you were unknowingly given something. The doctor can also check you for STIs and discuss pregnancy testing.

Most date-rape drugs are colorless, tasteless and odorless, so they can easily be slipped into a drink. Anyone who is drinking at a party – even if it's just soda – should keep her cup in sight at all times. And any girl who thinks she might have been raped should get to an emergency room as soon as possible – before changing her clothes or taking a shower - so the doctor could collect DNA samples for evidence.

My friend is turning in to a total slut! She hooks up with a ton of guys and I'm afraid she's going to get pregnant or catch an STI. How do I tell her to stop?

For starters, *slut* is such a harsh word. Some girls are just more sexually active than others, and if you criticize your friend for her choices, she'll just tune you out. Instead, approach her when she's alone and let her know you're concerned about her health and want to talk about it. Don't be judgmental, but tell her you want to make sure she's using protection *every time* she has sex. Ask her why she likes hooking up with different guys – maybe she doesn't get a lot of attention at home, or it helps to boost her self-esteem. If she realizes how much care about her, it may help her to curb her risky behavior.

I'm 16 and my boyfriend is 20. We've been dating for a year and we've talked about having sex. I feel like we're ready, but my friend to me it would be illegal! Is that true?

It depends. Every state in the US and every country in the world have an "age of consent," which is the legal age for having sex.

The age can be different for guys and girls and some places limit the number of years in age difference allowed between teen couples. To get an idea how much variation there is from place to place, check out ageofconsent.com - but understand that these kinds of databases are not kept up to date and the laws can change at any time. If someone over the legal age has sex with someone under the legal age, they could be charged with statutory rape. (Scary, huh?)

Since your parents *could* press charges against your boyfriend, talk to them and see where they stand. If that's not possible, at least talk to a trusted friend or relative but realize that if your parents don't approve of you having sex with him, he could get into legal trouble. Also, make sure you're discussed this with your boyfriend. Do you feel pressured to have sex to "keep up" with him because he's older? Is he willing to use protection *every* time? Laws or no laws, you need to be able to answer these questions before you even *think* about having sex.

All my friends talk about sex but honestly, I'm grossed out by the idea. Is something wrong with me?

Nothing's wrong with you! Just as we all get our periods at different ages, we all get interested in sex at different ages too. You're not weird at all – it's natural to be freaked out by the idea. Eventually, sex will become more important but until then, just be glad you don't have to worry about pregnancy, sexually transmitted infections, and all the other "fun" stuff that comes with sex. If you're really concerned, talk to your doctor to put your mind at ease.

My boyfriend and I started having sex a few months ago, but I've never had an orgasm. Am I doing something wrong?

First, let's talk about what an orgasm is. Technically, it's the climax of sexual excitement. For guys, this usually occurs with ejaculation but for women it's a little harder to define. You need to find out what is pleasurable for you and how you like to be touched. It's also really important that you feel comfortable with your boyfriend and you both want to have sex. If you are scared about your parents walking in on you or are worried about getting pregnant, you might not be relaxed enough to have an orgasm. And worrying about not having an orgasm can be distracting, stressful – and could prevent you from having one! So experiment with what feels good to you, communicate this to your boyfriend, use condoms to be safe, and above all, relax.

Condom Conundrums

I know you can get pregnant if the condom breaks during sex. But how can you tell if it ripped? Is it possible to feel it?

It's pretty hard to tell if a condom ripped – and even a tiny tear can make a condom ineffective in preventing pregnancy and sexually transmitted infections. Using lubricated condoms can reduce the chances of tears, but there are no guarantees. That's why you need to be prepared to face *all* the consequences if your contraception fails *before* you decide to have sex. And if you see even a small tear after using a condom, call your doctor and consider using Emergency Contraception if you're not already on the Pill or other hormonal method of birth control in addition to condoms.

Lately, condoms have been irritating my boyfriend's skin and I've heard that people can be allergic to latex condoms. Is this possible?

If your boyfriend has a condom problem, it's more likely to be a reaction to the spermicide on the condoms, not the latex in the condom themselves. Latex allergies are much more common in people who are exposed to the material over long periods – like doctors and nurses, who spend hours wearing latex gloves every day. Chances are he's reacting to the nonoxynol-9 spermicide added to many condoms to improve their anti-pregnancy effectiveness. Affected skin may be itchy or swollen, but it usually improves a day or so after exposure. Switching to condoms that are lubricated without spermicide may help. Condom packages will say whether or not the condoms have nonoxynol-9 added to the lubricant or not. Non-lubricated latex condoms are more likely to break, so a condom-safe lubricant would need to be used with them.

If your boyfriend is truly allergic to latex, his skin may get red and flaky where the condom has contacted his skin. This usually gets worse with every exposure, so if this is happening, he should see a doctor. Sometimes a mild steroid cream is needed to calm the skin irritation. If your boyfriend is diagnosed with a latex allergy, you can still practice safe sex. Used correctly, polyurethane condoms and the female condom (made of nitrile) protect almost as well as latex.

I've been with my boyfriend for two years and we're ready to have sex – but I don't want to get pregnant. I read that a condom has a 12 percent chance of breaking. Is that true? Is it better to use two condoms? I'm totally confused!

It's great that you're thinking about birth control before you and your boyfriend have sex. And you're right – though latex condoms are the best way to prevent STIs and HIV, they're only 88 percent effective in preventing pregnancy. That means that each year, 12 out of 100 girls who use only a condom during sex may get pregnant. The problem is people don't use condoms correctly – they're put on too late, or they break or slip off (including during removal after sex).

152

Using two condoms is definitely not recommended because it can actually cause the condoms to slip off easier. The best way to prevent pregnancy is to use something *in addition* to condoms. This could be oral contraceptive pills, Depo-Provera injections, a diaphragm, or spermicidal jelly/foam/suppositories. Spermicide may be the easiest choice because it's available in drug stores without a prescription. By inserting spermicide products inside you before sex, you can help kill sperm that may escape the condom.

Are the condoms in public restrooms safe? What about ones that glow in the dark? Are they less effective than regular ones?

There are so many types of condoms, so choosing one to use can be really confusing. So here's some info to help you sort it out. All *latex* condoms sold in the US – even the ones available in restrooms – should be safe because they're electronically tested for holes and weak spots before they are sold. So no matter what type of latex condom you use – super thin, extra strength, ribbed, colored, flavored, glow-in-the dark, etc - hey all meet the same set of standards for preventing pregnancy and STIs. However, there are some novelty condoms that are sold as a joke and clearly state on the package that they are not to be used for sex – so always check a condom's label.

There are few tips for better condom use: Check the expiration date (if there's only a manufacture date, don't use condoms more than 5 years after they were made). Make sure there are no rips on the wrapper – a torn package could mean a damaged condom. Use a condom every time you have sex.

Is it possible for a condom to get stuck up there during sex? This sounds really scary. How can I keep this from happening?

Yes, a condom can occasionally slip off and get left inside the vagina. But don't be too concerned - it's not going to get lost! You shouldn't have trouble retrieving it, although you might have to use a little fancy finger work. If you can't reach a lost condom, your doctor will be able to help you out. This kind of situation is not uncommon, so it's definitely nothing to be embarrassed about. And don't forget – *anytime* a condom slips off while you're having sex, you're at risk for getting pregnant and catching an STI.

Luckily, it's easy to prevent condoms from getting stuck inside you. Ask your boyfriend to feel for the rim of the condom during sex, and then hold the condom at the base of his penis when he pulls out. This will also reduce the chance of getting pregnant when using condoms.

Are two condoms better than one?

Only if you are going to have sex twice! Condoms are meant to be used one at a time, and if you layer them, they're likely to slip off or break from the friction of rubbing against each other.

If your concern is to prevent pregnancy or STIs, there are some better ways to do that. Keep condoms in a cool place and don't use them after their expiration date. When the time is right, put the condom on *before* you start messing around. Use spermicide with the condom to even further lower the chance of pregnancy. (You can buy spermicide in a number of forms – find the one you're most comfortable using.) Also, use plenty of water-based lubricant to keep intercourse friction free – not products which contain oil, which will melt the condoms.

What is a female condom? How are you supposed to put it on? Can it get stuck? Can a girl wear a condom and a guy wear a condom at the same time when they are having sex?

Female condoms are a bit tricky to use, but some women and their partners like them. They are thin PVC pouches with flexible rings at both ends. The ring at the closed end helps you insert it into the vagina. The ring on the open end stays outside the vagina during intercourse to keep the whole thing in place (and so it won't get stuck inside you). After sex, twist the condom's open end and pull it out. It lines the vagina completely, preventing any contact with a penis or semen, which is how it helps prevent pregnancy, STIs and HIV.

As for safety, female condoms are about 79 percent effective in preventing pregnancy. By comparison, male condoms are about 88 percent effective. These numbers are based on one year of "real life use," which takes into account the fact that female condoms are harder to use correctly. Like male condoms, female condoms protect against STIs but they may provide more protections against genital herpes and warts because they cover up more of the outside genital area.

Female condoms can be found at some drugstores (in the same aisle as male condoms) or online. They can only be used once and cost more than male condoms. Don't ever use male and female condoms together – they could break from rubbing against each other.

I've heard that using two condoms is way better than using one. This seems kind of tricky - is it really a good idea?

You'd think that more would be better, but this is definitely *not* the case. Condoms are made to be used one at a time. If you layer them, you actually increase the chances that one will slip off or break when they start rubbing against each other. The same goes for using a male and a female condom together. When used correctly, one condom is very effective in preventing pregnancy and STIs.

Since too much dryness or friction can cause a condom to break, choose one that's lubricated or buy a separate lubricant. Always choose lubricants that are water-based, not oil-based, to use with condoms. Using a spermicide with a condom will add extra protection against pregnancy. Spermicides come in jelly, foam, suppository or film formulations or choose a condom that already comes with spermicide (check the package). Then make sure your boyfriend puts the condom on right after he gets an erection to best protect yourselves from pregnancy and infections.

Guy Guidance

Recently, I head a bunch of guys at school whispering about wet dreams. I've heard of them, but I'm not totally sure what they are. Do girls get them too?

Starting sometime around puberty, guys begin to have wet dreams (the fancier name is nocturnal emissions). They're really just ejaculations that happen while asleep. When a guy's aroused – often by a sexual dream – his penis becomes erect and eventually releases semen. Most of the time, guys don't even realize they've had one until they find a wet spot on their sheets. We girls also get sexually aroused while we snooze, but because we don't ejaculate like guys do, there are no telltale signs in the morning, other than a little extra lubrication in the vagina. Lucky us!

What happens when I guy has an erection? Does it always mean he's turned on?

The inside of a penis is made up of spongy tissue. When a guy gets aroused (by thinking sexual thoughts or being touched) blood flows to the penis and fills up the holes in the tissue. The tissue gets firm when it's so full of blood, creating an erection.

But that doesn't necessarily mean that a guy is turned on at that moment. He could have been thinking about something a while ago (even if it was for only a moment) and still have an erection, because blood leaves the penis slower than it goes in. And sometimes, when guys are going through puberty, they can get erections for no reason at all – pretty embarrassing!

Female anatomy isn't that different – it's just not as noticeable. The clitoris and the labia also fill up with blood when girls have sexual thoughts, but since these parts are smaller than a penis, the change isn't as obvious to everyone around you.

What is the difference between circumcised and uncircumcised penises? I have no clue!

Believe it or not, besides looking different, there isn't much of a difference at all. In fact, both types of penises function exactly the same way. All baby boys are born with an uncircumcised penis, which has a fold of skin called foreskin that covers the tip of the penis. A circumcision is a surgical procedure that removes this overlapping fold of skin. Many parents opt for circumcisions soon after their baby's birth. It's done for cultural, religious, hygienic, and cosmetic reasons, but it's mostly done in the US, where more than half of all baby boys are circumcised. The rate of circumcision is lower in the rest of the world but recent studies showing that circumcision reduces the risk of cancer of the penis and some STIs may make it more popular in the future.

My guy friend says that he and his buddies, um, masturbate a lot. He says guys just physically have to do it. Is that really true?

Well, nobody, masturbates because they physically *have* to do it. Nothing horrible would happen to a guy if he didn't. The sperm will eventually just die inside his testicles. But it is perfectly normal for guys to masturbate. Many people – both guys and girls – masturbate because they like how it feels. It's that simple. And it is a totally natural thing to do, so you shouldn't think your friend is perverted or anything. There's nothing wrong or weird about you if you do or don't masturbate.

I know the first time is supposed to be painful for girls, but does it hurt for guys, too?

Intercourse can definitely be painful for men but it doesn't have anything to do if it is their first time or the thousandth. If a penis is bent suddenly or if testicles get hit or twisted the wrong way, guys definitely could experience some big pain down there.

Guys usually don't report that they had pain the first time they had intercourse, but that doesn't mean that it isn't true. The first time, they'd probably be more likely to get tangled up while messing around than they would after a bit of practice.

I hear girls joking about erections and ejaculation, but I don't know what either of those mean. Can you explain it? I feel so left out!

Erect means "straight" or "to build up," so it's kind of hard not to giggle when you hear someone say things like "stand erect" or "they plan to erect a skyscraper here." Erections are what happen when a man is sexually aroused and blood flow increases in the penis. The tissue inside a penis has holes like a sponge and, as blood fills up the area, the penis become firm, wider, and points up. Ejaculate means "to throw out," and ejaculation is the release of semen (fluid and sperm) from the penis. This happens at the end of the climax phase of sexual excitement. It can also happen while men are asleep during "wet dreams" – when sexually arousing dreams are so realistic that men's bodies react just as they would if those things were happening in real life.

This guy in school got an erection in the middle of class! Does this mean he's lusting after someone in class?

Not necessarily. Guys get erections on and off every day - and night - whether they want to or not. Lots of things can arouse a guy enough to cause blood to rush to his penis, from something he sees or thinks about for even a split second to the way his underwear rubs against him. If this sounds weird, think about what happens to *your* body when you're aroused – blood rushes to your pelvic area, causing your clitoris to swell and your vagina to become lubricated. But as girls we are lucky - the way we are built means the rest of the world doesn't have to know about what is going on in our pants!

Do guys always wake up in the morning with an erection? Why? Will it go away on its own?

Guys don't *always* wake up with morning erections (often nicknamed "morning wood") but they do sometimes. Yes, the erections go away by themselves. Most guys get erections on and off throughout the night while they sleep.

Erections are caused by an increased blood flow to the pelvic area, but no one knows exactly why they happen in the morning or during the night. Women also get periods of increased blood flow in their private parts several times a night. This occurs in both sexes because we're dreaming about sexual things. It's all normal and nothing to worry about.

This is embarrassing but here goes: What is the average penis size?

Penises come in a big range of sizes and shapes. If you look at a non-erect penis, you can't tell how big it will be when fully erect because the change in size can be a little or a lot. The average penis size is about 3.5 to 4.5 inches long when not erect and 5 to 7 inches when erect. The diameter of the penis also changes from about one inch when not erect to 1.25 to 1.5 inches when erect. But don't get out your ruler – these sizes are for grown men, not necessarily for guys your age.

What exactly happens when a guy gets an erection and how often does it happen?

Even though erections are commonly called "boners," there are no bones inside a penis. The inside of a penis is made up of spongy tissue. When a man gets aroused by thinking sexual thoughts, blood flows to the penis and fills up the holes in the spongy tissue. The tissue gets firm when it's so full of blood, creating an erection. After a period of no sexual arousal or after an orgasm, the blood flows out the penis and it is no longer erect.

Female anatomy isn't that different, the change is just less noticeable. The clitoris and the labia also fill up with blood when a woman has sexual thoughts, but because these parts are smaller than a penis, the change isn't as dramatic.

My new boyfriend just told me he's not circumcised. First of all, I'm not really sure what that means. And now I'm wondering: Is it dangerous to fool around with him?

There is basically no difference between a circumcised and uncircumcised penis, other than the obvious one – the way it looks. Circumcision is the removal of the foreskin, the hood-like piece of skin at the tip of the penis. Some guys refer to it as being "cut" if they are circumcised or "uncut" if they're not. Uncircumcised men have a slightly higher chance of getting cancer of the penis, but most doctors agree that the difference is too small to recommend circumcision for all men.

In the US, over half of boy babies get circumcised soon after birth but it's much less common in the rest of the world. Parents usually decide to circumcise their sons for cultural or religious reasons, because it's easier to not have to clean under a foreskin, or if the baby's father is circumcised.

I'm not ready to have sex, but when my boyfriend and I fool around and then stop, he says it physically hurts him. Is that really painful for guys?

The old "blue balls" excuse, huh? What he's complaining about is pelvic congestion, commonly called blue balls. But that name isn't accurate, since no part of his body actually turns blue! During sexual excitement, blood flows to the genitals, causing guys to get erections. If a guy doesn't ejaculate, the blood hangs out there for a little while and slowly returns to the rest of his body. While it's there, it could cause a dull ache or discomfort, especially in the testicles which feel heavier than usual. But it isn't actually *painful* and it's not dangerous. Because not ejaculating is the problem, masturbating or just waiting for the erection to do away will help. Some men use this excuse to pressure women into having sex, but don't be fooled. Only you can decide when you are ready.

About the Author

Ilana Newman, MD graduated from the University of Arizona with three bachelor's degrees in four years. Before starting medical school at the University of Arizona, she did an internship at MTV in New York, where she worked on the alternative music show 120 Minutes. This experience fueled her interest in adolescent health issues. While in medical school, she found some interesting ways to combine her media experience with medicine, including medical school electives with the medical news unit at the CBS Evening News and KROQ's Loveline show.

Dr. Newman chose to specialize in family medicine instead of pediatrics because most adolescent health problems (sex, drugs, eating disorders, acne, sports injuries, depression, etc) are not problems common in little kids. She completed her family medicine residency at Beth Israel Medical Center in New York and became certified to use acupuncture in New York State. Afterwards, she did a fellowship in adolescent medicine at the Mount Sinai Adolescent Health Center in New York. She appeared in health segments on the Oxygen Network and had a monthly column in Twist magazine. Later, she wrote and hosted a daily online medical news show for doctors.

Many years later, Dr. Newman did another fellowship in hospice and palliative medicine at the University of Miami. She currently treats patients with advanced cancer and other life-limiting conditions, helping to manage the symptoms from their disease or treatments. She is a voluntary assistant professor in family medicine at the University of Miami, where she helps teach the acupuncture course for physicians.

Resources

To find an adolescent medicine physician in your local area, check your health insurance company's list of providers under pediatric specialists.

Another place to find an adolescent medicine physician is a teaching hospital with a pediatric residency program. All pediatric residents are required to do one month of adolescent medicine training, so each of these programs should have an adolescent medicine specialist on staff.

Other adolescent medicine resources:
1) Mount Sinai Adolescent Health Center -
http://www.mountsinai.org/patient-care/service-areas/adolescent-health-center
2) Society for Adolescent Health and Medicine (SAHM) –
www.adolescenthealth.org

www.ingramcontent.com/pod-product-compliance
Lightning Source LLC
Chambersburg PA
CBHW021828020426
42334CB00014B/540